boosting
your energy

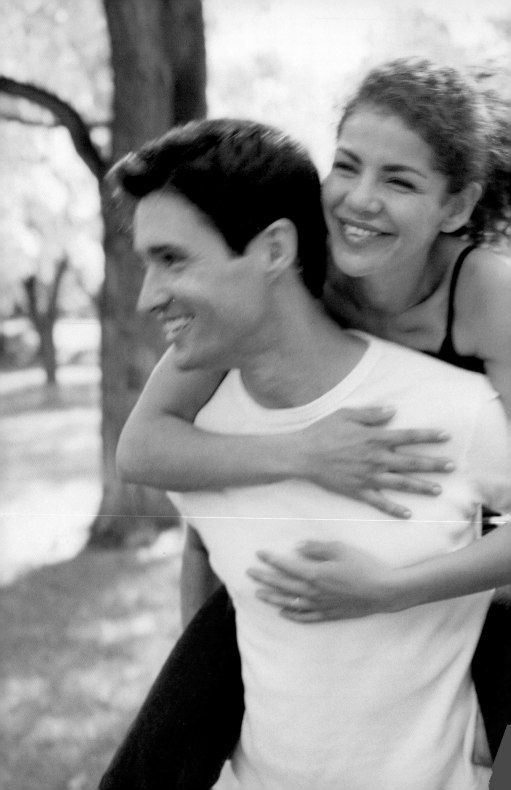

boosting
your energy

through conventional and alternative methods

hilary boyd

Consultant: Dr. Len Saputo

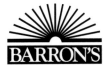

First edition for the United States, its territories and dependencies, and Canada published in 2003 by Barron's Educational Series, Inc.

First published in Great Britain in 2003 by Mitchell Beazley, under the title *Options for Health: Boosting Your Energy.*

Mitchell Beazley is an imprint of Octopus Publishing Group Ltd, 2-4 Heron Quays, Docklands, London E14 4JP

All inquiries should be addressed to:
Barron's Educational Series, Inc.
250 Wireless Boulevard
Hauppauge, New York 11788
http://www.barronseduc.com

International Standard Book No.: 0-7641-1902-8

Library of Congress Catalog Card No.: 2003102212

Typeset in Futura and Folio

Printed and bound by Toppan Printing Company, China
9 8 7 6 5 4 3 2 1

Executive Editor	Vivien Antwi
Executive Art Editor	Christine Keilty
Project Editor	Peter Taylor
Design	Nicola Liddiard
Copy Editor	Rona Johnson
Picture Research	Emma O'Neill
Proofreader/Indexer	Jane Gilbert
Production	Alexis Coogan
Medical Consultant	Dr. George Lewith

Picture Credits

Front cover Bananastock; 2 Corbis/LWA-Stephen Welstead; 12 Image State/AGE/Stuart Pearce; 15 Octopus Publishing Group/H. Verrinder; 21 Corbis/Steve Prezant; 26 Getty Images/Eric Jacobson; 29 Octopus Publishing Group/Mark Winwood; 31 Bananastock; 35 Image State/AGE/Ben Welsh; 38 Getty Images/Patrick Coughlin; 40 Pascal Goetgheluck/Science Photo Library; 45 Photodisc; 47 Bananastock; 51 Corbis/Rob Lewine; 57 Robert Harding Picture Library/Dr. Dennis Kunkel/Phototake NYC; 61 Image State/AGE/Jonnie Miles; 66 Corbis/Ariel Skelley; 71 Alfred Pasieka/Science Photo Library; 75 Corbis/Hans Georg Roth; 79 Corbis/Ted Horowitz; 80 Bananastock; 84 Octopus Publishing Group/Jason Lowe; 92 Photodisc; 95 Octopus Publishing Group/Stephen Conroy; 100 Octopus Publishing Group/Gary Latham; 105 Corbis/Pete Saloutos; 107, 112 Corbis; 117 Corbis/Jim Cummins; 120 The Art Archive/Private Collection/Dagli Orti; 123, 127 Corbis; 128 Getty Images/Elizabeth Simpson; 133 Corbis/Digital Art; 134 Image State/AGE; 139 Photodisc.

Publisher's note: Before following any advice or exercises contained in this book, it is recommended that you consult your doctor if you suffer from any health problems or special conditions. The publishers cannot accept responsibility for any injuries or damage incurred as a result of following the advice given in this book.

contents

foreword

We all want our lives to be filled with good health and unlimited vitality. Every year consumers spend billions of dollars attempting to buy these items as though we were purchasing a refrigerator. And yet, the foundation for a life filled with abundant energy is built on just a few basic lifestyle principles that are available to most of us at very low cost.

There are certainly times when our bodies break down for reasons beyond our control. We have all known people who have suffered from illness even though the way they live their lives seems ideal. While there are strategies from a wide range of disciplines that promote healing, the style in which we live our lives—our lifestyle—remains the most powerful tool that supports healing and the development and maintenance of optimal health. Factors such as eating a healthy diet, getting enough rest, exercising regularly, living a life with minimal stress, consuming sufficient high-quality water, finding meaningful purpose in our lives, and taking time to enjoy our lives, all stimulate the body to initiate its own innate inner healing mechanisms. This is simple to understand, but in today's world it is not always so easy to put into action.

In the interest of saving time, we generally speed through life, often forgetting that life is a process, not a destination. In our haste, life may become more of a chore than an interesting exploration. We have invented fast food that is now filled with everything besides real food—it is highly refined, processed, often stored for long periods, and has many synthetic chemicals added for a variety of reasons having nothing to do with good nutrition. Our lives are filled with stress—we live in the fast lane passing by everything except for the immediate goal in front of us. We don't take enough time to smell the roses. We spend too little time living in the moment. We don't connect with nature. And, many of us are so tired at the end of the day that we don't take time to enjoy exercise or our relationships.

What we have done is to create hundreds of thousands of new chemicals that have created a serious problem with pollution. We are the only species on the planet that has had the "wisdom" to pollute our food, water, and air. And, what may be even worse, many of us have taken on materialistic values that are centered on accumulating money and wealth, and that distract us from the most important purpose in our lives—our relationships.

As our fast-paced, space age lives zip past us at what seems the speed of light, all too often many of us miss out on the simple important basics that provide us with high-energy levels and vibrant health. The first step in creating a healthy lifestyle requires having a clear understanding of what these basic principles are. *Boosting Your Energy* explores these premises and offers practical solutions that anyone can learn. It also goes beyond mainstream medical approaches and explores exciting new and popular complementary and alternative strategies that are practical and do-able. You can gradually incorporate each principle, one by one and at your own pace, into a lifestyle that will build good health.

While this book addresses the physical and biochemical causes for low energy, it also probes deeper into emotional and spiritual perspectives. It takes the whole person—body, mind, and spirit—into account as it explores the causes and provides solutions for the many faces of fatigue. And, it blends the best therapies from the East and West, and from conventional and alternative medicine. This integrative style provides the unique opportunity for each person to select those special therapies that are appealing and feel right to incorporate into his or her life. It encourages and empowers each of us to take responsibility for our own healthcare, and do it with confidence.

Boosting Your Energy is also written for those interested in prevention and wellness. We don't have to wait until we become fatigued or get sick before taking action. Being proactive to preserve our health and vitality makes sense if we're to get all that we want out of our lives.

Energy is what makes the universe work. It is also what makes our body, mind, and spirit work. Without this precious and powerful gift life could not exist. Everything we do and everything that happens all around us requires energy—everything.

Len Saputo, M.D.

introduction

We are living in a high-speed world, and we need maximum energy to enjoy it. But the pressures of modern life can easily drain our feeling of well-being, with the result that many of us are finding energy and vitality in very short supply. This is because the harder we drive ourselves, the less time we have to look after ourselves, so we live a quick-fix life: fast food, too many stimulants, too little sleep, no exercise, and too much stress. Added to which our bodies are constantly under attack from air pollution, water pollution, noise pollution, electronic pollution, and pollutants in food.

Vitality

It's little wonder that we have gotten used to feeling tired, and that tiredness has become one of the most common complaints of our age. Too many of us wake up tired because we have slept poorly, then drag ourselves through the day with no energy for anything else beyond our essential routine, be it sport, social life, or a hobby. Our energy levels support survival, not vitality.

Finding our energy

But we can find our energy again. We can nurture our body back to health, and function at the peak of our potential, with the result that we wake up bright eyed and bounding with vitality, set to face the day with a sense of pleasure, not dullness.

To do this we have to address the problem in all areas of our life: our physical body, our mind and emotions, our spirit, and our daily environment. We have to find a balance in the way we eat, sleep, work, exercise, and relax our bodies. This is because if any of these elements of our way of life are out of kilter, our energy levels tumble.

Making the change

This book's first aim is to help you to understand your energy levels and identify the areas in your life that may be causing you to feel tired and lacking in vitality. The book then offers a range of positive lifestyle alternatives to help increase energy levels.

It's never easy to change your life, but it is definitely worth it if the reward is increased vitality and enthusiasm for life. We are often reluctant to start a healthier regime because we think it involves giving up what we enjoy, but for most of us it is more of an adjustment than a radical change, based on replacing toxins with energy-boosting nutrition, learning to deal with stress, and getting our bodies moving.

Complementary therapy

The second half of the book explores the complementary therapies that might help, in conjunction with these lifestyle changes, to increase vitality. These include therapies such as acupuncture and reflexology, yoga, tai chi and Pilates to increase suppleness and inner strength, meditation to calm the mind, and herbal remedies to boost the immune system.

What this book suggests is an informed, realistic commitment to energy boosting rather than an all-out, obsessive health kick. It involves first eliminating the energy-depleting elements in your life and then finding a regime of diet and exercise that will suit you, and, most importantly, that you can enjoy and maintain in the future.

Once you have adjusted your life patterns and your energy begins to rise, you will wonder how you survived that old couch-potato way of life.

So get some energy and start living!

How the tabs work

Following the sections on specific conditions and health problems in Part One is a series of colored tabs. These relate to the color-coded sections in Part Two of the book where you will find more information on the therapies most likely to be appropriate for treating a particular condition.

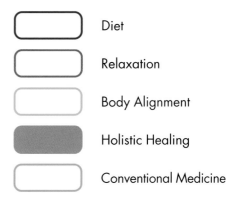

Diet

Relaxation

Body Alignment

Holistic Healing

Conventional Medicine

setting your goals

Unfortunately there is no energy standard to which we should aspire. We can test our blood, we can scan our brain and body, but we cannot accurately measure our energy level. So each of us has to decide whether we are happy with the amount of energy we have for our individual way of life.

How much energy do we need?

Because we are all different, even if there were an energy standard it would be almost impossible to define the right amount of energy for each individual. Added to that, our energy needs are always changing, depending on what stage of our lives we have reached.

But it would appear that most of us are not happy with our energy levels. We may get through most of our life without serious disease, yet we would not be categorized as ill, nor would we feel exactly bounding with energy. In fact a lot of the time we feel just "a bit below par."

How is lack of energy affecting your life?

Human beings are notoriously resistant to change. Our daily commitments put constraints on us, it's true, but if a change to a healthier way of life is suggested most of us have a string of excuses a mile long as to why it won't work for us.

We hear ourselves complaining that, for instance:

- "I don't have time to exercise."
- "I have to eat what the family eats."
- "I can't avoid alcohol at a business lunch."
- "My partner smokes, so I can't give it up."

So it is important to take a long, hard look at your way of life and pinpoint exactly how your lack of energy is affecting your life. Think back over your day. Do you have the energy to do what you want without feeling exhausted? Are you constantly irritable because you are tired? Are your relationships with family and work colleagues suffering? If so, there is no reason to believe that nothing can be done to improve things.

In short, there are simple, commonsense ways to increase the energy you need to survive your particular day, whether it involves coping with the demands of family life or dealing with stress in the office.

Two steps to more energy

Increasing your energy is a two-step process. The first step is to cut down and gradually eliminate some of the habits that are contributing to low vitality.

These will vary from individual to individual. Some will need to cut down on fast food, some on stimulants such as alcohol and cigarettes, and some to reduce the stressful elements.

The second step in the process is to build up the nutrient and exercise levels that will nurture your body back to peak performance.

Be realistic

Once you have identified the reasons for wanting to increase your energy and vitality, and then concentrated on what might be at the root cause of your low energy levels, the next task is to set realistic goals so that you can bring about the desired change in lifestyle.

No improvement happens overnight so it is essential, if you are going to succeed, to find an energizing regime that can be accommodated realistically within the structure of your life.

Your program is unlikely to work if you rush at it and decide to detox, give up smoking and alcohol, and take up strenuous exercise all at once. So when you are deciding what steps to take, make sure the program you choose is one you can see yourself sticking to, not just for the next few weeks, but as an ongoing lifestyle plan.

To backslide is only human, but we are less likely to do so in any major way if we are happy with our commitment.

Read on and find out what your choices are for the diet and exercise plan that suits you best; the essential changes you need to make in order to achieve the health and energy needed to enjoy life to the fullest.

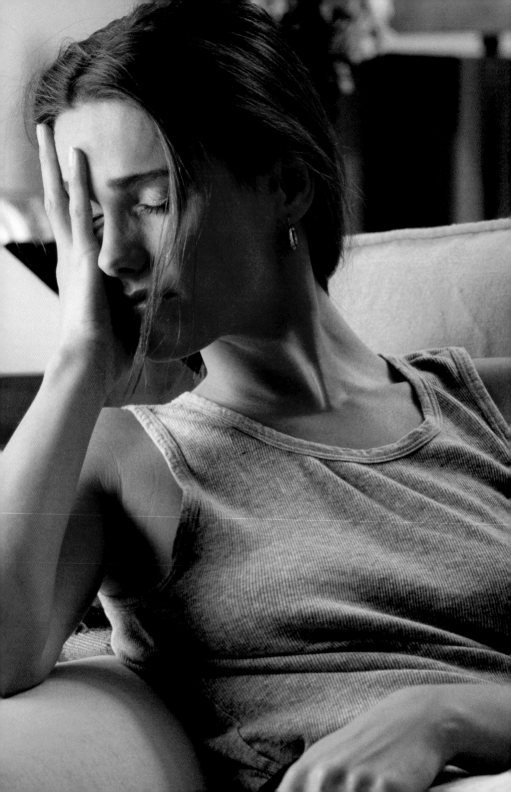

under-
standing
the problem

Before embarking on an energy-boosting program, it is important to understand about the source of your energy and the ways in which you deplete it: the input-output equation.

Despite significant advances in public health – safer water, immunizations, dry housing – our bodies are still exposed to pathogens, the microbes in our environment that cause disease. We push ourselves ever faster to keep up with the speed of modern life and expect too much from our bodies. We pile in the toxins as if we were waste disposal units, then complain that we have no energy. This section explains the energy equation and pinpoints where you might be going wrong.

understanding your
energy
levels

Energy production is a very complex affair that involves all the body's systems working together to give us the vitality we need to go about our daily life. Our whole body, down to the smallest cell, is one huge "energy organ" and therefore a large number of factors exist that can influence our energy supply.

The energy equation

It would be much simpler if there were one single energy gland in the body that produced our energy, just as the thyroid gland produces thyroxine, then when we were feeling particularly enervated we could test our blood for low energy levels and apply the appropriate remedy. But, because the whole body has to work to produce energy, the source is difficult to pin down. Unless we are ill, we eat, sleep, walk, talk, and work without collapsing from exhaustion.

All the body's systems rely on a regular and adequate supply of air, light, water, and the nutrients we get from our food, but the key to our basic energy level is the balance of energy input to energy output.

Metabolism The way we turn food into energy is complex. Put simply, our basic energy comes from this sequence of events:

■ We breathe in oxygen from the air.

■ Oxygen is transported around the body via the bloodstream – all cells and organs rely on oxygen. Without it the body ceases to function within minutes.

■ We drink water; water accounts for around 70 percent of body weight and is vital for organ function. We get at least half the water we need from our food.

■ We eat food, which includes water, carbohydrates, fat, protein, minerals, and nutrients.

■ The digestive system breaks down food so that the body can absorb it.

■ The by-products of digestion – sugars, fatty acids, amino acids – are then either used immediately for energy output, or stored for use at another time.

Ways we use energy

■ Even when we are sitting completely still, we are using energy simply to maintain our body functions – such as breathing, blood circulation, and core temperature. This minimum energy expenditure is known as the basal metabolic rate (BMR).

An adult's daily BMR uses an average of 20-25 kilocalories (84–105 kilojoules) per kilo of body weight (1–1.2kcals per minute). The BMR is related to body mass, and so is slightly lower in women and as we age, as there is less body mass. It falls when we are asleep.

■ We expend energy when we eat, and the body utilizes ingested calories by converting them into usable forms or stores them.

■ Energy is expended constantly by all the movements our bodies perform, even ones we are unaware of, such as fidgeting, scratching, crossing our legs.

■ The greatest energy expenditure is from exercise, either from work or sport. This last expenditure of energy is variable, depending on our way of life.

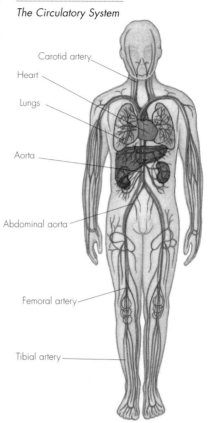

The Circulatory System

Carotid artery

Heart

Lungs

Aorta

Abdominal aorta

Femoral artery

Tibial artery

One of the keys to high energy is balancing energy input with energy output.

Vital energy

Beyond the basic input-output energy equation, our vital energy comes into play. This can be best described simply as "vitality," that extra component that makes our day a pleasure, not merely a grind, and is reliant on more than the metabolism of our food.

The human body can stay alive on basic minimum rations but to have vitality we have to achieve harmony in all our body systems. This includes the quality of the food we eat, the way we exercise our bodies and, importantly, the state of our psyche, i.e., how happy and fulfilled we are, and how we deal with the stresses of everyday life. For many of us this is the Holy Grail, the elusive factor we crave but cannot pin down, the difference between just functioning and really living.

In Eastern philosophy this is known as the mind, body, spirit connection, and is believed to be influenced by the universal energy flow, or *qi*, which is said to be present in all living organisms. Some styles of complementary medicine are based on the principle of maintaining the free flow of *qi* around the body.

Lethargy

Problems of tiredness and lethargy arise when body-energy is disrupted for some reason and becomes out of balance. This can have many causes.

Weak immune system Disease is a major cause of energy imbalance and it is also thought that energy imbalance is a cause of disease. Any illness, even a minor cold, will sap our energy.

Pain Being in pain, whatever the cause, produces body tension, which in turn strains our system and drains our energy.

Stress Stress in itself is not bad; it is how we deal with it that affects our energy.

Poor diet Our bodies need fuel, but many of us are giving ourselves the wrong type of fuel. Although many conventional doctors don't agree, there now appears to be a clear association between allergies and food intolerances and low energy. And, too many high-sugar foods for quick-fix energy make blood sugar levels unstable. This can cause energy slumps and irritability. A poor diet can also mean unwanted weight gain, which puts an added strain on the body.

Addiction Excessive use of all drugs from alcohol to prescription medicines put all the body systems out of balance, resulting in a false energy fueled only by more of the addictive substance.

Body pollution Pollution, smoking, and toxic impurities in food can all increase toxin levels in the body; this puts a strain on the organs and can drastically reduce energy.

Antibiotics It is thought that antibiotics may, in some cases, disrupt the balance of intestinal bacteria leading to overgrowth of the yeast *Candida albicans*. This can give rise to symptoms such as low energy.

Sedentary lifestyle To keep our bodies strong and in balance we must move around. Stamina and flexibility, which directly affect the functioning of all our body organs and therefore energy levels, are achieved only through exercise.

Depression People who are depressed have been shown to have reduced brain activity. This affects their mood and lowers their general energy levels.

Negative outlook One of the biggest energy zappers of all time is a negative outlook on life. Someone with a negative outlook will be forever looking for the insult, the downside, the ulterior motive, and this negativity will promote anxiety, which will promote stress, which in turn will drain valuable energy supplies.

Basically when any of these factors interfere with the smooth working of the body, some of the mechanisms that regulate our system begin to break down and our energy levels plummet. We will discuss internal and external factors in more depth in the chapters to come, and the more we understand how we make our energy supply and how we deplete it, the more likely we are to be able to avoid the pitfalls and put in place some long-term strategies for boosting our energy not just in the short term, but as part of our daily way of life.

Should I worry?

Low energy levels are both a warning of disease – we often feel tired and listless in the days before we develop even a minor infection – and the result of disease. So how do we know when low energy requires medical attention?

This section outlines additional symptoms to look for and the possible underlying causes.

The most common causes of low energy are stress, poor diet, lack of exercise, and toxins in food, water, and air, so attention to these areas can be of great value.

But there may be some underlying medical problem that should be addressed. The most common medical causes of fatigue are anemia, diabetes mellitus, hypothyroidism, depression, or viral infections such as flu or the Epstein-Barr virus, which causes infectious mononucleosis.

Adverse drug reactions, particularly to those drugs that help lower the blood pressure, may also drain energy.

When it's not just tiredness...

Low energy is a universal symptom of an imbalance in the body. There are many different reasons why this happens. But reassuringly, our bodies have a great capacity to restore these imbalances, and medical attention is not usually required.

And most diseases that require treatment have a variety of additional symptoms apart from low energy, which will help to identify them.

Anemia This is when hemoglobin, the oxygen-carrying element in red blood cells, is low.
Symptoms include: faintness, pallor, and shortness of breath on mild exercise.

Diabetes mellitus There are two types of this condition:
Type 1 commonly starts in childhood and is more severe; the treatment involves insulin replacement.
Type 2 usually starts in adulthood and can be controlled by diet and exercise. It has increased alarmingly in the Western world and the reasons for this are not yet established, but it is thought to be strongly connected with obesity.
(See box on p.19.)

DIABETES MELLITUS

!

This is a serious condition where the body is unable to properly metabolize sugar, either because there is not a sufficient supply of insulin, or because the body does not respond to the insulin available. The symptoms include:

- *Excessive passing of urine*
- *Excessive thirst and a dry mouth*
- *Lack of energy*
- *Weight loss, despite eating*
- *Blurred vision*

If you are experiencing some or all of these symptoms, please consult your doctor at once.

Hypothyroidism This is when the thyroid gland, which regulates body temperature and the speed at which the body metabolizes fuel (see p. 70), does not produce enough of the thyroid hormone, thyroxine.

Symptoms include tiredness, cold hands and feet, intolerance to cold, unusually dry skin, thinning hair, constipation.

Depression Sufferers often complain first of tiredness and lack of energy.

Symptoms include low mood, lethargy, difficulty in sleeping, lack of interest in life, poor concentration. (See p. 74.)

Viral infection Any viral infection, such as flu or glandular fever, can induce low energy both during, and for some weeks after, the infection.

Symptoms include swollen glands in the neck, lethargy, a sore throat, fever, and severe and ongoing low energy and fatigue. Symptoms vary according to the virus. If you experience a fever, which is when your body temperature goes over 38 degrees Centigrade, (100 degrees Fahrenheit), you should drink plenty of cool fluids – mineral water is ideal for this – and take an over-the-counter painkiller such as acetaminophen. If the fever persists or keeps rising, consult your doctor.

the
mind-body
connection

It seems obvious that our mind and body are inextricably connected. It is clear that one influences the other, and that the smooth functioning of all human beings relies equally on both.

Yet, extraordinarily, until quite recently Western health philosophy had made little, if any, concession to the mind-body connection. Perceptions, fortunately, are changing.

The holistic approach

Our energy levels are related to our overall health – body, mind, and spirit. We cannot have vitality without this. This holistic approach to health, which looks at the whole body, has been a tenet of Eastern healing philosophies such as Ayurveda – the Indian system of healing – and traditional Chinese medicine for thousands of years. But Western medicine over the last 150 years has been carried away by science and technology, developing ever more sophisticated drugs and surgical techniques at the expense of treating the patient as a whole person. We were in danger of losing the mind-body connection altogether.

Advances in technology are immensely valuable in medicine. We can now replace someone's heart, vaccinate the world against smallpox, and treat killer diseases such as malaria, typhoid, and AIDS. It would be foolish to dismiss modern medicine and claim that conventional treatments, for example chemotherapy drugs, have no value. People are more than just the sum of their body parts.

Find the key to vitality

Unfortunately, because of this high-tech health philosophy, many of us in the Western world have come to see good health as something to which the doctor holds the key. We have allowed the "absence of illness" to be our standard for good health, and this attitude does not address the quality of our health and energy when we are not feeling ill. So we can proudly claim that we "haven't seen a doctor in years," but during those years we may not have felt exactly bright eyed and bursting with vitality. In order to regain our vitality we must take responsibility for our health, and the most effective way to do that is to reinstate the holistic approach and start seeing the mind-body connection as the key to improving overall vitality.

What do we mean by our "mind?"

We talk about the mind-body connection, but what exactly do we mean by our "mind?" The brain is the control center of the body. On a subconscious level – meaning we don't have to think about it – through what is known as the autonomic nervous system, messages from the brain regulate all our body functions, such as breathing, heart rate, muscle tone, digestion and hormone balance, our sight,

Good health is more than just the absence of illness; it is the harmony of mind and body.

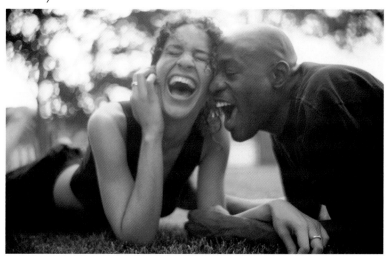

hearing, taste, and our response to pain. But as well as these subconscious brain messages triggering mechanisms in the body, there are other, less easily definable but equally important, components of every human being: our thoughts, emotions, and spirit. And it is these, and their interaction with the autonomic nervous system, to which we are referring when we talk about the mind-body connection.

Danger response

For example, imagine you are walking along a road and you are suddenly confronted by a mugger with a knife. You are terrified and your subconscious brain triggers the "fight or flight" response (see box below), which gives you the chance to escape and save your life. You do escape, but your conscious mind is traumatized by the event, your thoughts and emotions still making you frightened.

And although your body is no longer being threatened, these anxious thoughts about danger trigger the same response in your body that the actual physical danger did, in that more stress hormones are being secreted into your bloodstream, making your heart rate and breathing faster.

If not dealt with, this could develop into an anxiety disorder, which in turn might put a strain on your physical body through tension and the effect of high levels of stress hormone, which in turn might compromise your immune system, making you more vulnerable to disease.

FEAR: FIGHT OR FLIGHT

- We are frightened
- As a result, the pituitary gland in the brain secretes a higher level of a hormone called adrenocorticotrophic hormone (ACTH)
- This ACTH immediately acts on the adrenal glands to secrete the stress hormones adrenalin, noradrenalin, and cortisone
- Adrenalin and noradrenalin increase the heart rate and respiratory rate and shunt blood flow from the intestine to the muscles and cortisone mobilizes glucose, so that we are fired up enough to cope with any life-threatening emergency

Happiness and health

As we can see, body and mind, and the effect that each has on the other, are not independent. Body and mind are inseparable; they do not exist as separate entities.

A relatively new science called psychoneuroimmunology (PNI) investigates the interconnection between psychology, the nervous system, and the immune system. One PNI study found that a group of medical students under exam stress showed a decline in the number of T-lymphocytes or T-cells (the cells that fight off viruses and cancer) in their blood.

Dr. Patch Adams, the famous American doctor and healer, was one of the most recognized members of the conventional medical profession to acknowledge the link between happiness and bodily health. Believing that joy and laughter are as important as drugs, he began his work 30 years ago by visiting sick children in the hospital where he worked, clowning around to make them laugh.

Influencing the mind If the mind can affect the body, then the body can affect the mind. For instance, when we take a stimulant such as coffee, we find our mind initially more alert, but if we drink too much we become wound up and irritable. A low blood sugar causes tiredness and short temper. Pain puts us in a bad mood, and we feel pain more when we are in a low mood, much less if we are happy.

Energy and the mind-body connection

Our energy levels, like our health, are directly influenced by both mind and body. It is important to stress the word "both," as there is a lot of New Age nonsense that implies that feeling well is merely a process of thinking well, that health and energy are the preserve only of the mind. This is dangerous thinking.

We can, however, exert considerable control over our bodies; slow, deep breathing causes the nervous system to slow the heartbeat. People who meditate regularly find it much easier to relax and cope with stress.

We can support our quest for better energy levels with a positive mental attitude and mind-calming techniques, especially if balanced with exercise and nutrition. What we are seeking is a balance between mind and body, a holistic approach to energy boosting that benefits the whole person, and gives all the systems in the body the fine-tuning they need to function optimally.

lifestyle influences on energy

Now we're coming to the crunch. This section looks at how we might be sabotaging our chances of high energy by some of the lifestyle choices we have made. And although it may seem easier just to keep on drinking all that coffee, or downing all that fast food while we stamp our feet in protest at the thought of denying ourselves "treats," it is important at least to know how all these toxins with which we so casually bombard our bodies might be contributing to the problem. And although there are some things we would undoubtedly be wise to change, this is not about making us lead a boring life of misery and denial. Not at all; in fact it's the reverse. It's about treating ourselves well and improving the quality of our life. So that we will feel the best we can.

diet and weight

Food is our fuel, so the quality of what we eat is a vital factor in our levels of energy. But diet has become a major 21st-century obsession, with a great deal of confusing advice. For many of us food is no longer a pleasure but has become a source of guilt and personal conflict. It is time that some common sense was brought to the subject.

What is a "good" diet?

What we eat and the way we eat it is reflected in the way we look. People who eat poor, unnourishing food over a long period are likely to have low energy levels, and dull skin and hair. They might have weight problems, and may eventually succumb to diseases such as heart disease, liver disease, diabetes, and various forms of cancer, which may be preventable with proper nutrition.

So what is a "good" diet?

Just as it is impossible to set an energy standard that is appropriate for everyone, so it is impossible to have a one-diet-fits-all scenario.

Even the word "diet" has worrying connotations these days, with many people trying to lose weight using a variety of fashionable diets on which they are expected to eat only protein, for example, or raw food, or a caveman diet. Most of these diets are hardly compatible with a normal life.

Good, healthy nutrition depends on finding the right food plan for your age, height, build, and metabolism, and one that fits in with your lifestyle. It should consist of food that you enjoy and that you are not just forcing yourself to eat; it should be varied, and it should be simple, using fresh, unprocessed food wherever possible.

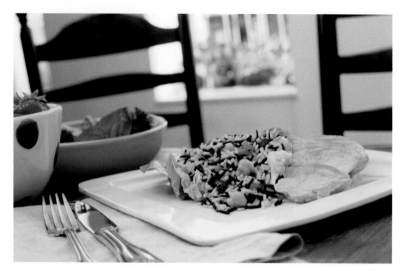

Modern food science can sometimes be alarming, but you can't go wrong with a diet containing fresh, unprocessed food, including lots of fruit, vegetables, and whole grains.

Healthy eating guidelines

Food science is advanced enough these days for the experts to have reached some consensus on healthy eating guidelines. We know enough about the constituents of foodstuffs – the vitamins, minerals, fats, proteins, and sugars – to say that, for instance, carrots contain vitamins A and K, thiamine, folate, calcium, iron, manganese, phosphorus, and zinc, and to understand what benefits these vitamins and minerals have to our bodies.

And it has been generally agreed that a healthy diet consists of a balance of around 60–70 percent complex (i.e., wholegrain) carbohydrates, 20–25 percent protein, and 10–15 percent fat, preferably unsaturated, accompanied by plenty of fruit and vegetables, and between 1.5–2 quarts (1.5–2 liters) of water a day. (Vitamins and supplements are discussed in detail under "Diet" on p. 90.)

New research

Almost every day, however, new research is published that challenges or modifies this current wisdom. One of the most significant new ideas to emerge recently is the idea of categorizing food by the glycemic index scale, which measures how much a certain food affects our blood sugar levels. (The glycemic index scale is discussed in more depth under "Diet" on p. 88.)

By cutting down on foods that release sugar into the bloodstream too fast, it is thought we can avoid the high levels of insulin and unstable blood sugar levels that give rise to low energy and erratic mood swings.

Other research is more alarming. For instance, oily fish such as salmon and mackerel – long considered nutritionally valuable – worryingly is now thought also to contain high levels of mercury and dioxins, picked up from industrial effluents flushed into the sea and entering the food chain. And the baked potato – touted for years as one of the healthiest of foods we could eat – is not only a high glycemic index food but also, apparently, when it is cooked at a high heat contains the carcinogen acrylamide in its skin.

However, much of what you read in the press reporting food scares is not yet backed up by sufficient research to confirm initial suspicions.

CHECK YOUR BODY-MASS INDEX

The statistics are alarming. Obesity is now thought to be the fastest-growing health threat in the developed world, especially among children. Heart disease, Type 2 diabetes, stroke, and some cancers are all more likely to affect people who are obese. Too much extra weight puts a strain on all the body systems.

Obesity is now calculated by measuring our body-mass index (BMI), the ratio of height to weight: a normal body mass is between 20–25, overweight is between 25–30, obesity is over 30.

To check your own BMI:
■ Measure your height in feet (meters), and multiply the result by itself, i.e., squared
■ Measure your weight in pounds (kilograms)
■ Divide your weight by your height in feet (meters) squared

Nurture your digestive system

We can all survive on a meager diet lacking in a proper variety of nutrients, it is true; unfortunately, large sections of the world's population do just that every day of their short lives. But if we want high energy we must help our digestive system to function at maximum efficiency, because digestion is key to turning food into fuel.

It's no good just eating what is deemed to be healthy food, if we are preparing and eating it in the wrong way or in inappropriate quantities, or if our system is intolerant to it because of sensitivities or antibiotics, or factors such as too much alcohol or caffeine are sabotaging the absorption of nutrients.

When any of these factors are present, the digestive system, although it is receiving healthy food, is not able to process the essential nutrients and deliver them to the body organs. We discuss this in more detail in the "Diet" section later in the book (see p. 83).

Treat food with respect

Casual and erratic eating habits are one of the major problems of modern life. The concept of the "meal" has gone, and in its place is a fast-food, fast-eating culture, where food is no longer respected. This trend is in part responsible for the current epidemic of obesity, and it definitely contributes to low levels of energy.

We eat a breakfast bar on the bus going to work, then grab a coffee when we get there. We pop out for a sandwich and a bag of chips at lunchtime, and eat them at our computer. We get home exhausted and starving, and down half a bottle of wine to help us relax, then shove a frozen dinner into the microwave, which we gobble in front of the TV.

Or we don't eat at all during the day, just drink coffee, then consume all the day's calories in one huge meal in the evening.

Does that sound at all familiar?

So yes, we have eaten, but the food has been random and the process not savored. By eating this way we are not nourishing our bodies to achieve the most beneficial balance of nutrients, and our energy can suffer.

Food should be a pleasure. We should set aside time to enjoy eating it as a sensory, relaxing, enjoyable event.

We can't find the time? Yes, we must!

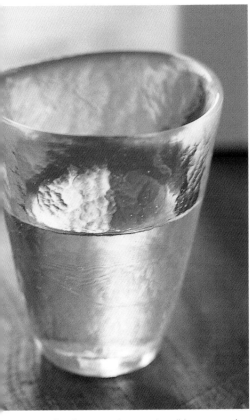

Water, water everywhere ... or at least it should be. Try to drink 1.5–2 quarts (1.5–2 liters) a day.

Dehydration

Food is one thing, but what about water? We think of dehydration as a state that only happens to those who get stuck in the desert, but in fact most of us are suffering from low levels of dehydration every day of our lives and this alone can make us tired and lacking in vitality.

We need around 2–3 quarts (2–3 liters) every day to replace the fluid lost by the functioning of our bodies; we lose fluid just by breathing, sweating, excreting urine and feces.

This is not nearly as alarming as it sounds because we obtain around 1 quart (1 liter) of that fluid from the food we eat, but we do still have to make up the rest of what we need from drinks.

Some people go through the entire day, however, without drinking water other than in drinks containing stimulants such as coffee, tea, cola, or alcohol, all of which are not only dehydrating, but also diminish our body's ability to flush toxins from the system.

Assessing our diet

So if we are to have high energy we have to take a careful look at what and how we eat. It is not only a matter of balancing calorie input with calorie output, but whether we are eating wholesome, high-energy food in appropriate quantities, whether this food is suitable for our lifestyle, age, and digestion, how we take our meals, how many toxins we add to our diet, and whether we drink enough water.

the
importance
of exercise

Exercise, in conjunction with a healthy diet, is the cornerstone of high energy. No one who leads a largely sedentary life will be able to achieve his or her maximum energy potential.

We need to move our bodies to increase the circulation of oxygen and nutrients to vital organs, to strengthen and mobilize our muscles and to burn off stress chemicals.

Make the first move

We were not designed to lead sedentary lives. Modern technology has contributed to this immensely. Motorized transport – buses, planes, cars, escalators – and labor-saving devices – everything from vacuum cleaners and washing machines in the house to leaf clearers and electric hedge clippers in the garden – have reduced to almost nothing the need for us to exert ourselves, so it is essential to fill that gap with regular exercise.

How fit? This need not be a heavy-duty regime; it depends on what you enjoy and the level of fitness you want to achieve. Age and health status will dictate how far we can push our bodies. This means getting our bodies moving if we are to function at the peak of health and vitality.

How does exercise affect your energy?

Strength, flexibility, endurance, burning stress hormones and calories, and a strong heart all result from regular exercise. Exercise is not, as many of us think, just about building six-pack abdominal muscles. But there is one muscle, the heart muscle, that needs to be particularly strong, and the only way to strengthen it is to exercise regularly and aerobically, which means increasing your heart rate by exerting yourself.

It works like this: a good supply of oxygen and nutrients are essential for optimum body-organ function. They are delivered via the circulation, by the pumping of the heart. When you exercise, heart rate increases and you breathe faster. You not only take in more oxygen, but the oxygen and other nutrients in the blood are circulated efficiently to meet the increased demand on organ and tissue function.

Increased circulation from exercise means:

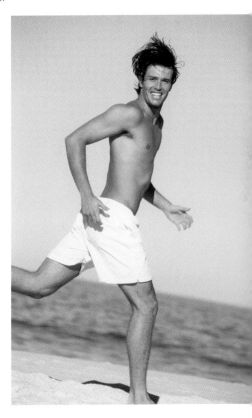

■ Your brain will be more active, which results in increased vitality.

■ Your liver will eliminate toxins more efficiently such as external pollutants, stress hormones, and damaging cholesterol.

■ Your muscles will become stronger so your skeleton will be better supported.

■ Your immune system will be enhanced making you less vulnerable to illnesses.

■ Endorphins and enkephalins – mood-enhancing brain chemicals – will be released.

■ You burn more calories.

■ You strengthen your heart and improve bone density, helping to protect against the likelihood of future heart disease and osteoporosis.

Without exercise we will never reach our maximum energy potential.

Body image

The way we look is important to how we feel. We needn't aspire to being super-models; "look" means overall image: posture, weight, skin, hair and nail quality, and the clearness of our eyes. As we discussed earlier, mental health is tied inextricably to physical health (see p. 20). If we look good we feel good and vice versa, and this gives more confidence and less anxiety. Exercise and a healthy diet dramatically improve how we look and how we feel. We are less likely to be overweight, we will have better posture, skin and hair will be healthier, and levels of vitality and self-esteem will be higher.

Exercise for life

We know it's good but the very word "exercise" still strikes terror into many hearts. It doesn't have to mean discomfort, self-sacrifice, and boredom. Remember that bossy exercise video – now gathering dust in the corner – or the gym that, despite the fortune you paid, you couldn't bring yourself to visit? You remember failure.

If the thought of going through that humiliating process again seems like too much effort, you are missing the point. Regarded as a competition or a punishment it will never become an integral part of your daily life. Try seeing exercise as the new member of the family. Sometimes it will annoy you, sometimes it will seem too tiring, but it is also a joy and, most importantly, exercise will be here to stay.

Get moving

Getting moving at first can be hard. But you don't have to start with a full-on commitment, especially if it is a while since you last did any exercise. Don't think about your muscle tone yet; just start to wake up your body. Get moving so the circulation begins to flow more efficiently. The benefits will quickly inspire you to do more. It sounds simple doesn't it? And it is, once you've gotten started.

Most of us would like to exercise. Getting started is the problem. One of the reasons we view the process with suspicion is that if we haven't exercised for a long time, the effort it takes even to walk upstairs is huge and physically uncomfortable.

Tips to help you begin

■ Treat exercise like learning a new skill. Start at the beginning, focus, and realize you won't be proficient overnight.

■ Take it at your own pace; it's not a competition, you're not going to be tested, so what's the hurry? You risk injury if you push yourself beyond your capabilities.

■ Decide on an exercise you really enjoy; don't just opt for the current trend, and take your age, weight, health, and previous experience into account.

■ Be realistic. Are you really going to get up at 6 A.M. in the winter?

■ Find someone who is at the same stage of fitness and arrange to exercise with them – perhaps your children! Join a dance class, take a walk, or swim together.

■ Start small. A 10-minute stretching program you can do at home, plus a brisk half-hour walk three times a week is a good start if you are unfit. Then you can gradually increase as your strength and stamina improve.

■ Think "Move!" Walk to the next bus stop, take the dog for longer walks, walk upstairs, don't drive the car for short distances. Walk briskly, stand tall, and breathe deeply. Feel the energy firing through your body.

■ Buy a comfortable pair of walking shoes, and carry more fashionable ones.

■ Exercise outside. Fresh air is just as good for adults as it is for children.

■ Don't forget to drink lots of water.

None of the suggestions above is hard, but all require a commitment. Turn to p. 104 for guidance about specific types of exercise and their relative benefits, find one to suit you and your lifestyle, and "get moving."

stress
factors

"I'm stressed-out" has become one of the favorite catchphrases of the 21st century. Not all stress is bad; we need a challenge, but if we lose control and become swamped by the pressure of modern life, then stress begins to take its toll on energy and health. It's important that we face up to the factors that create too much stress.

How does stress affect your energy?

Stress is one of the biggest causes of low energy. Human beings have a very sensitive response to anxiety; it is a vital survival mechanism. Our brains respond to the various stresses our day brings – an important meeting, a performance, an argument with a partner – by triggering our adrenal glands to supply the necessary amount of stress hormones (adrenalin, noradrenalin, and cortisone) that give us the energy boost we need to cope. In extreme circumstances, this same mechanism might save our life.

This is how it should be. But if your body is experiencing constant, unwanted stress, the ongoing secretion of low levels of stress hormones will begin to build up within the tissues. And if you don't address your stress problem these raised levels will, in time, adversely affect all your body systems. This can contribute to a host of conditions from depression to heart disease, eczema, stomach ulcers, panic attacks, palpitations, headaches, irritability, nausea, mood swings, sleep disturbance, loss of libido, aches and pains, and osteoporosis.

Good stress, bad stress We live in a very stressful world, there is no doubt about that, but every generation has stress. Now the problem is speed: fast travel, fast communication, fast food. We have lost our ability to slow down. The pressures of a fast-paced lifestyle are certainly villains in our fight against stress, but how well we cope with those pressures is really the vital factor.

Without some stress many of us would never get out of bed. The sort of stress that motivates us is healthy, exciting stress. It is an exam, a deadline, a new job that drives us forward, and if we are coping well with a particular challenge this healthy stress can have a good impact on energy levels.

Bad stress usually happens when we are not enjoying these everyday challenges. We are not controlling our life; our life is controlling us.

External and internal stress factors

External factors are the stressful life events themselves. There are the negative ones, such as bereavement, divorce, moving, losing a job, contracting a serious illness, or being a victim of crime, and also social circumstances such as poverty and isolation. And there are the positive factors, such as changing jobs, taking an exam, making a speech, or running a race. These events can happen to all of us over a lifetime and it would be foolish to think we can avoid them.

The internal factor is equally, if not more, important as a contributor to stress; it is the way in which each individual deals with stressful, external life events. How we deal with stress is a very personal process; some people are naturally better at it than others. For some, stress is classified as having someone to supper; for others it is running an international corporation.

Everyone is faced with stress – it is how we deal with it that matters, and some are better at coping than others.

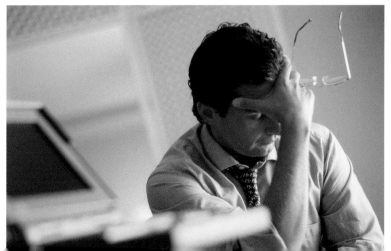

But stress can only be quantified by the person suffering from it. You might think your friend has an easy life, yet to him it seems very stressful because his coping mechanisms are poor.

Self-induced stress

Whether we are good or bad at dealing with stressful life events, most of us also contribute to our anxieties by adopting stress-inducing lifestyle habits. For instance, people who can't say "no" find that everyone makes claims on their time.

We drink excessive amounts of tea, coffee, caffeinated drinks, or alcohol. We smoke. We eat poorly and erratically. We don't exercise. We find it difficult to admit to our problems and ask for help. We don't plan ahead.

If all this seems familiar, then you have to accept that you are not helping your cause. You are living on chemical energy and reducing the internal energy levels that might help you cope.

Added to which we may feel stress about our image. Are we thin enough, svelte enough, pretty enough, and are we dressed fashionably enough? Are we successful enough or rich enough?

Unconscious stress

The external world is also an environmental stress machine. Although most of us do not realize it, the pollution in food, water, and the air, the noise of traffic both on the ground and in the air, and the sheer press of people all contribute to stress.

Then there is the strain on our bodies from all the toxins we are often unaware

ANGINA

Angina occurs when there is constriction in the blood flow leading to the heart. It usually happens on exertion or with stress and is characterized by a pain that spreads up into the throat and down the arm, usually the left, starting with a heavy constricting sensation in the center of the chest, like a steel band around the heart. If you experience this pain, seek medical help immediately.

that we are absorbing, such as food additives and preservatives, pesticides, dioxins, mercury, lead, and acrylamide. All these pressures use up valuable energy and can effectively reduce our vitality.

Managing unwanted stress

While we may not be able to eliminate all of these stress promoters from our lives, we can do much to minimize their effect on us with good diet, exercise, and relaxation techniques. But the first and most important step is to recognize and acknowledge that we have a problem.

We have got so used to being wound up, rushing through our days with no time to think, that many of us have begun to accept that high anxiety is just a part of life. But that is a dangerous way to think. Take a look at your life and ask yourself these questions:

- Do you sleep well?
- Do you wake up in the morning rested and alert?
- Do you have time to yourself when you can relax and do your own thing?
- Do you laugh a lot?
- Do you avoid compromising either your work or your home commitments?
- Do you feel healthy and free from aches, pains, and minor illnesses?
- Do you ever have time when your cell phone is switched off, not counting when you are in the movies or at meetings?
- Do you find it easy to keep your temper?
- Do you have the energy for a social life and a sex life?
- Do you enjoy at least one freshly cooked meal a day, at a table?

If you have answered "no" to four or more of the above, you are badly in need of some stress-reducing techniques.

Stress and energy Chronic stress wears your batteries down. First you slow down and function less efficiently, then you stop altogether. But by recognizing stress and facing up to your contribution to it, you can soon begin to recharge those depleted body batteries.

We look at ways to plan this in the second half of this book.

lack
of sleep

Sleep disturbance is one of the most common causes of low energy. Without adequate sleep we function poorly, and if the sleep shortage is chronic we can become ill. Everyone can go a couple of nights without much sleep, and catch up successfully later in the week, but if we suffer regularly from broken nights, then our energy levels and health will plummet.

Why do we sleep?

Oddly enough, scientists don't really know the specific reasons why our bodies need sleep. Cell regeneration is not affected by lack of sleep. The nervous system does require rest but the chemical and biological mechanisms for why this should be are not yet clear. However, it seems reasonable that we should want to switch off our conscious thought processes and rest our bodies every day.

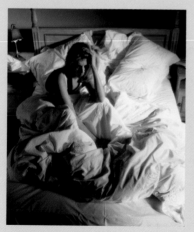

If our natural sleep pattern is interrupted too often all the body systems are weakened. We can feel cold, tired, listless, irritable, depressed, our digestion becomes sluggish, our heart rate erratic, and if the sleeplessness becomes chronic we become more vulnerable to ill health.

If you don't sleep on a regular basis your energy levels will begin to suffer.

Quality not quantity This changes over our lifetime. Babies sleep most of the time; old people and those who lead a sedentary life need less. Some people function well on only a few hours a night – Mrs. Thatcher famously on four hours – while others religiously take their eight hours but remain tired during the day. The quality and our specific needs, rather than the number of hours, of sleep are more important. A few hours of good, deep sleep are more beneficial than tossing and turning all night. But worrying about sleeplessness is the worst thing you can do, as it will probably keep you awake even longer.

Reasons for sleeplessness

■ **Stress and anxiety** cause an overproduction of stress hormones, which can disrupt sleep.

■ **Stimulants** such as caffeine, nicotine, and drugs such as cocaine and amphetamines will disturb sleep.

■ **Eating habits,** for instance a heavy meal late in the evening, will play havoc with digestion and blood sugar for some people.

If you boost your insulin too high, then later in the night it may plummet and trigger the release of adrenalin, which could disturb your sleep. Some people will get the same result if they don't eat enough in the evening.

■ **Lack of exercise** can keep you awake. Exercise tires you out, allows stress hormones to be burned off, and releases endorphins, the body's natural opiates.

■ **Medical conditions** such as depression, hyperthyroidism, sleep apnea (see box below), side effects of prescription drugs, and withdrawal from sleeping pills can disrupt sleep.

OBSTRUCTIVE SLEEP APNEA

This is when your breathing stops when you are asleep for up to 10 seconds, five or more times an hour. It occurs when the upper airways become blocked due to relaxation of the tissue around the pharynx.

Symptoms include disturbed sleep, loud snoring, poor concentration, daytime sleepiness, and morning headaches. The condition is exacerbated by smoking, drinking, and excess weight. If it is severe it can cause life-threatening heart rhythm problems.

addiction

We do not think of ourselves as addicts. But the truth is that many of us are virtually addicted to habits such as smoking and drinking alcohol. And if we want to raise our energy levels these habits need to be modified because they zap our vitality, disrupt sleep, and put an unnecessary strain on our body systems.

Altered states Alcohol, tobacco, and recreational drugs temporarily alter our mental and physical state, which when we are under stress and low in energy is just what we want – a short-term lift to help us relax and forget our worries. Alcohol is a sedative, although initially it reduces inhibitions and raises confidence. Nicotine acts as a tranquilizer on smokers, giving them an immediate feeling of relaxation as

The effects of mind-altering substances on the brain can now be measured by sophisticated electronic scanning.

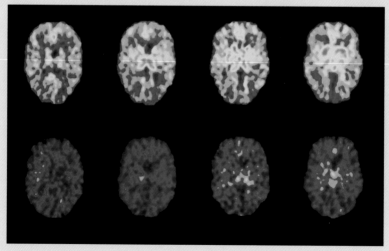

their nicotine craving is temporarily assuaged. Recreational drugs such as cocaine are stimulants; marijuana is a relaxant. But far from making us feel better, these drugs can create dependence and if used regularly and in inappropriate amounts wreak havoc with all the body's systems. In short: address the underlying lifestyle problem that is draining your energy, rather than turn to chemical energy.

Alcohol

Much pleasure is derived from sipping a good glass of wine or a cold beer with friends. And taken in moderation, with plenty of alcohol-free days in between, drinking less than five glasses of wine a week should not diminish your energy.

However, if you get drunk it takes the liver at least two days to recover, and the more you drink the longer it takes for your body to return to normal. Because alcohol increases sweating and urine production it causes dehydration, which puts added strain on organ function, and disrupts sleep. Taken long term and in excess, alcohol contributes to potentially fatal heart, liver, and brain disease, and to accidents.

Because alcohol, particularly red wine, contains fungus and chemical additives, it may exacerbate the symptoms in anyone with a blood sugar imbalance, or a sensitivity to yeast – *candida* – overgrowth, for example, which is thought to be a major cause of low energy. (See "Diet" section on p. 83.)

DO YOU HAVE A DRINKING PROBLEM?

■ Do you ever feel guilty that you drink too much?
■ Have other people commented on how much you drink?
■ Do you drink at times of the day when other people don't, for example, first thing in the morning?
■ Has alcohol interfered with your work or home life because of hangovers, bad temper, or accidents?

If you have answered "yes" to any of these questions, you should consider changing your drinking habits and, if need be, seek help. Groups such as Alcoholics Anonymous have a high success rate.

The most important point about alcohol is that it is alarmingly easy to become dependent without realizing it, especially at times of stress. (See box on p. 41.) Those who find it difficult to limit their intake to the occasional glass may do better to stop drinking altogether to allow the body to detoxify and raise energy levels.

Cutting down Most of us simply need to be aware of how much we are drinking and take steps to cut down if necessary. List all the alcohol you have drunk over the past week. If you find you are drinking regularly or heavily, or feel you need alcohol to relax or to sleep, then it's time to consider getting help to address the problem.

Start by having one day each week when you don't drink. Alternate each alcoholic drink with a glass of water. Try refusing the first drink of the evening, say you'll have one later, and once over the initial craving, you may find you don't want that drink at all. The difference it will make the next morning will spur you on.

Nicotine

Smoking tobacco is straightforward. Don't do it. There is no upside. Tobacco smoke contains literally hundreds of chemicals, including nicotine and tar, many of them carcinogens. These chemicals damage all the body systems, making the smoker susceptible to cancer and heart and respiratory disease. Smoke irritates the lining of the airways and inflames the lungs; this increases mucous secretion and decreases lung capacity, which results in less available energy-giving oxygen.

Smoking encourages wrinkles, promotes early menopause, and depletes the body of vital vitamins and minerals. The RDA for vitamin C is increased by 35 mg a day for smokers, for example. And nicotine is highly addictive. Enough said.

Giving up Smokers finding it hard to quit can try many different supports, from hypnosis to nicotine patches, helplines, and books. Ask your doctor for advice. But give up and enjoy better energy levels and a healthier and a longer life.

Drugs

We are well aware of the dangers of illegal, recreational drugs such as cocaine, ecstasy, and heroin, but many of us are less clear about the potential for becoming addicted to over-the-counter or prescription medicines. This form of dependency is said to be 10 times greater than the problem of illegal drug abuse. A pill is available for almost everything these days, from heartburn to headaches, bacterial infections to sleeplessness. For many of us, having a health problem means we expect to take some sort of pill. And if the medication is prescribed by a doctor or pharmacist we may assume it is safe and fail to check its potential side effects.

Beware dependency The three classifications of drugs most likely to cause dependency are:
- **Opioids,** or drugs taken for pain that contain morphine or codeine.
- **Benzodiazepines,** or central nervous system depressants, usually taken for sleep or anxiety disorders.
- **Stimulants,** which are less commonly prescribed than they used to be, but are still used to treat attention deficit disorder in children, and narcolepsy, a rare sleep disorder.

These drugs are generally safe if taken over a short term and as prescribed, but people do become addicted to medicines, unaware that they have a dependency problem until it is well established.

Kick out toxins Substances such as those mentioned here have the potential to create high levels of toxicity in your body. It is never easy to break a habit, particularly if that habit involves physical dependency. It is important to find whatever help you need to wean yourself off excessive, energy-depleting substances if you are to significantly improve your health and vitality. You can't underestimate the negative effect smoking, drinking, and drugs have on your long-term well-being.

DRUG ADDICTION

Warning! If you think you might have a problem with long-term use of a particular drug, don't attempt to come off it on your own. Seek medical help. Your doctor will probably prescribe a gradual reduction in the dosage, and treatment for any unpleasant withdrawal symptoms you might be experiencing.

environmental
pollution

We live in a sea of pollution. Without realizing it we are assailed by thousands of chemical pollutants and radiation. But in addition to these specific toxins, we also pollute our lives with noise and clutter. The body has learned to adapt to a certain extent, but the strain on our systems shows up in depleted energy levels.

Air pollution

Carbon monoxide, from incomplete fuel combustion in central heating boilers and car engines, impairs the function of oxygen-carrying red blood cells. High levels of nitrogen oxides, ozone, and sulphur dioxide make us vulnerable to respiratory diseases such as bronchitis, and may trigger asthma attacks.

As we breathe in air, cilia – tiny hairs that line the upper airways – filter dust and small particles of dirt, the lungs expel some pollutants in exhaled air and via the cough reflex, and many toxins are processed and excreted via the liver and kidneys.

Protect yourself

Exposure to pollutants is part of modern everyday life, but there are steps that can be taken to minimize exposure.

- Make sure your central-heating ducts are cleaned regularly.
- Cut down time spent in heavy traffic; avoid taking exercise near busy roads.
- Minimize use of aerosol sprays and turn away from the spray where possible.
- Make your home, office, and leisure areas no-smoking zones.
- If you use chemicals at home or work, follow recommended safety instructions.

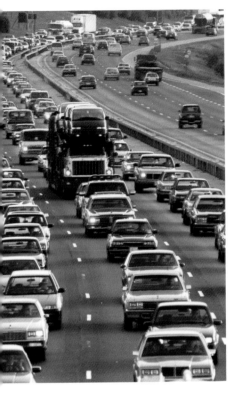

We love our cars, but they don't contribute to high energy levels.

Food pollution

Estimates for the number of toxins found regularly in the food we eat vary from 5000 to 250,000: from organo-phosphates used in pesticides to mercury and dioxins in fish. These are thought to contribute to problems such as cancer, allergies, and hyperactivity in children. Try to eat organic produce and avoid processed food.

Radiation

Some forms of radiation are still not satisfactorily monitored or regulated. We are exposed regularly to food irradiation, electromagnetic waves from overhead power lines, TVs, and cell phone antennas. We are subjected to microwave emissions from cell phones and ovens, and emissions from computers and visual display units (VDUs).

Excessive radiation can cause cancer, miscarriages, and birth defects, but electronic equipment such as computers and VDUs are also thought to contribute to headaches, eye strain, and tiredness. Limit the time you are exposed to unprotected sources such as VDUs or cell phones.

Clutter and noise

Avoid clutter and disorganization; they do not enhance energy. Losing things or forgetting appointments causes stress and wastes or drains your energy. Noise also causes stress and stress uses up energy. Traffic, planes, piped music, cell phones, stereos, crowds, and mechanical equipment all contribute to high levels of noise. Spend some time each day surrounded by silence.

relaxation

Relaxation is the remedy for stress. It allows body and mind the space to regenerate. It is vital to have regular periods of relaxation programmed into our day, yet how many of us really know how to relax anymore? Today's busy-busy world tends to equate relaxation with laziness, but relax we must if we are to maximize our energy.

Balance at work and play

We work ever longer hours in this competitive world, although the jury is out as to whether we actually accomplish more. Many people pride themselves that they are always on the go, but by denying themselves time and space to think, time to "be" rather than "do," they are neglecting the elements that enhance spiritual development, such as intuition, creativity, and perspective on life.

Our bodies need to get rid of the stresses of the day. Hours hunched over an office desk, the commuter crush, lugging heavy shopping – all are routines that create muscle tension and fatigue. But if at home you slump in front of the TV, your body never has the chance to move freely and let go of that accumulated tension.

We all need to find a balance in life between work and play. Take a moment to assess how much time is spent each day relaxing and doing your own thing.

Switch off

There are many different ways to relax, from sports or gardening to yoga or a scented bath. What is important is that you have chosen it, that you are doing something you want that gives you pleasure, and allows you to switch off from the stresses of the day.

Socializing with close friends is a good way to relax. Sharing your thoughts with others stimulates the mind, boosts self-esteem, and sheds light on problems. We all need company.

Make time to contemplate

As well as pleasurable pursuits we also need contemplative time. This is time when we can connect, away from worldly distractions, with a universal consciousness that is bigger than ourselves.

If we don't manage to do this, either through a spiritual philosophy or religion, we risk rushing through a life that has no meaning beyond the material. And a spiritual component in our lives has been shown to enhance the body's healing mechanisms; it is the third element in homeostasis, the mind, body, spirit balance. Meditation is ideal for this. (See the "Relaxation" section on p. 98.)

Organize your life

They say that hell is paved with good intentions, and most of us procrastinate when it comes to tasks we don't enjoy. But putting things off is not relaxing, because the guilt and worry that we have not done something just creates another stress.

How often have you finally done something you've been dreading, and found yourself flooded with relief and surprise that it wasn't as bad as you had been anticipating?

So the next time you say to yourself "I'll do that later," stop, take a deep breath, and do it now.

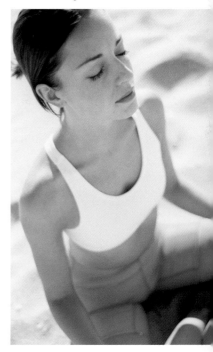

Go out more

Most of us spend much of our day indoors. This means we have no access to sunlight, fresh air, and the natural world. Nature soothes us and takes us away from the pressures of our daily routine.

Go for a walk, sit on a bench, look up at the trees, feel the sunlight on your face, and fill your lungs with fresh air.

This is a perfect way to spend some of your lunch hour, or to wind down after work.

Life is not all about "doing" – we must all find time to just "be."

medical causes for low energy

We all feel low in energy and lethargic at times; this is natural. We might have a particularly heavy work schedule or suffer a personal upheaval. But as well as our lifestyle habits there are medical causes for low energy, and it is important to recognize the difference.

We feel tired when we are ill, even with a head cold; it is a warning sign that something is wrong, but persistent or severe tiredness needs medical attention. Tiredness and lethargy are symptoms associated with chronic pain, and illnesses such as cancer, blood disorders, allergies, hormone imbalances, and infections. This section outlines diseases associated with low energy, but if you are worried about your health, consult your doctor.

chronic pain
syndrome

Chronic pain is thought to affect at least 10 percent of the population, and it often has a devastating effect on those who suffer from it. It is most commonly caused by muscle, joint, or nerve damage, and is seen in diseases such as cancer. But whatever the cause of chronic pain, the result is almost inevitably low levels of energy.

Pain: nature's alarm system

Without pain we might not know when we are ill or injured. Pain may be the main reason for seeking medical help. So although we fear pain, it serves a purpose. Acute pain makes us snatch our hand away from a flame, and it alerts us to a wound or an infection.

When acute pain becomes chronic Most of us experience acute pain fairly frequently, when we bang our head, fall over, or cut ourselves, and we tolerate the pain that goes with the healing process. But occasionally pain persists long after the normal healing process should have been completed. This pain does not serve either as a warning sign or to trigger the healing response. It just hurts. And pain that seems to have no end in sight is much harder to bear.

The impact of chronic pain We cannot see pain, nor can we feel someone else's pain, and there is no single pain experience, so it may be hard for others to understand our pain. But pain exhausts, disturbs sleep, and can prevent us from carrying on with normal life. Work, relationships, sex life, fitness level, and weight may become disrupted. To help cope with chronic pain there may be a tendency to take up addictive habits, such as heavy drinking or taking excessive amounts of painkillers, all of which alter mood and behavior. So after a while not only the pain must be dealt with, but the isolation, depression, and addiction it engenders.

The mind-body connection

There is a strong mind-body perspective in the way we perceive pain. Pain triggers both a physical and an emotional response. Both consciously and unconsciously we can either magnify pain, or diminish it.

For example, you have burned your hand. The burn is throbbing and very painful and you feel sorry for yourself. Then a friend calls with tickets for your favorite band. You become suddenly less aware of your pain; it hurts just as much but you push the pain consciousness to the back of your mind.

This unconscious response can be harnessed in pain management using techniques such as meditation and visualization.

Common causes of chronic pain

Apart from injury, there are many conditions that feature pain as a symptom, but the most common causes of chronic pain are damage to muscles in the back, arthritis, shingles, and headache.

Back pain Lower back pain is said to affect over half of the adult population at some time every year. It is usually caused by injury to the joints, ligaments, and muscles that support the spinal cord, and can be triggered simply by bending or twisting, or by lifting a heavy object inappropriately. Other common back problems include slipped disks.

Symptoms include pain felt in the lower back or neck that radiates into the legs or arms; it can be brought on or aggravated by stress or emotional tension.

Treatment Conventional treatment might include rest, painkillers, and physiotherapy. Complementary alternatives could include acupuncture, chiropractic, or massage. With back pain, however, prevention is better than cure: improve your posture, take regular exercise, make sure your office chair supports the small of your back, follow sensible lifting guidelines, wear comfortable shoes, and avoid stress.

Rheumatoid arthritis This is a condition in which the synovial membrane, which lines the joints, becomes inflamed resulting in swollen, stiff, painful, and eventually deformed joints.

The condition can affect any joint but usually starts in the hands and feet and progresses, attacking both sides of the body at the same time. There may be remissions when the sufferer remains symptom free for months or even years.

There are many techniques you can use to help manage or alleviate chronic pain.

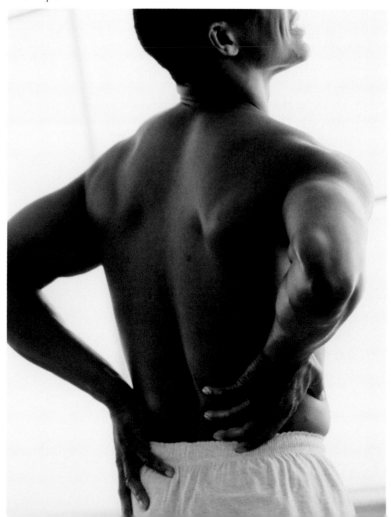

Symptoms include tiredness and poor appetite accompanied by painful, swollen joints, morning stiffness, and small painless nodes on some joints.

Treatment Conventional treatment may include nonsteroidal antiinflammatory drugs (NSAIDs) such as aspirin and ibuprofen (Advil), or antirheumatic drugs that slow or stop joint pain. A splint may be worn to support the joint and help prevent deformity. Complementary treatment may include dietary advice, acupuncture, reflexology, homeopathy, or naturopathy.

Osteoarthritis This is the gradual wearing away of the cartilage that protects the ends of the bones inside the joints. As the cartilage disappears, the bone may develop bony spurs called osteophytes and the joint may become progressively stiff, swollen, and painful. It is important to remember that some degree of osteoarthritis is usual as we age and that it is not necessarily painful or debilitating. Its causes are not yet clearly understood.

Symptoms include pain that is worse on movement, stiffness when inactive, swelling around the joint, enlarged joints, restricted movement, cracking when the joint bends.

Treatment Conventional treatment may include: acetaminophen or NSAIDs for pain, corticosteroid injections into the joint to reduce pain and inflammation, or joint replacement. Complementary therapies could include chiropractic, acupuncture, exercise, food supplements such as cod liver oil, glucosamine sulphate, chondroitin sulphate, and green-lipped muscle extract.

Migraine This is a fairly common condition. Attacks can occur several times a month. No one knows exactly what causes migraine, although it may be brought about by dilated blood vessels in the brain, or as the result of chemical and electrical disruption in the brain. Contributory factors include familial predisposition, stress, lack of sleep, and foods such as cheese, red wine, and chocolate.

Symptoms include a severe throbbing pain, made worse by movement, often on one side of the head, often preceded by visual disturbances such as bright flashes or blurred vision, acute sensitivity to light and sound, and nausea and vomiting.

Treatment Conventional treatment may include drugs to prevent migraine, drugs to relieve migraine once it's started, and painkillers. Complementary treatment could include chiropractic, aromatherapy, relaxation techniques, or Bach flower remedies.

Preventive measures to avoid a migraine include avoiding stress, strobe lights, and foods that might trigger an episode, and maintaining a regular sleep pattern.

Shingles Caused by the chickenpox virus (herpes zoster), shingles appears as a painful, blistered rash that develops along the path of a nerve, usually on the face, chest, or abdomen. Chronic pain may result from the continued neuralgia, or nerve pain, after the condition itself has disappeared.

Symptoms include a painful blistered rash, tiredness, fever, headache, and ongoing neuralgia.

Treatment Conventional treatment might include antiviral medicines and painkillers. Complementary treatment could include acupuncture and intravenous vitamin C.

Pain clinics

Pain management is a relatively new but growing area of medicine. Pain clinics are set up with a multidisciplinary team of specialists qualified to look at all the different aspects of pain. Once the team has defined the cause or causes of the pain they will prescribe a plan to help you to either eliminate, reduce, or cope with it.

Treatment can include drugs, surgery, counseling, relaxation techniques, and complementary therapies such as acupuncture, either in isolation or combination.

BEWARE NSAIDS

Warning. Nonsteroidal anti-inflammatory drugs (NSAIDs), such as aspirin and ibuprofen can damage the stomach lining. This can lead to gastritis, ulcers, gastric bleeding, and kidney failure. This can happen without warning.

When using NSAIDs make sure you take them with food, and consult a doctor if you are required to take them repeatedly, especially if you are over the age of 60.

illnesses

As with pain, the other symptoms of disease are warning signs, which we ignore at our peril. Sometimes symptoms can be vague and insidious, as with diabetes and some forms of cancer, but being alert to changes in our body, such as persistent low energy, and what this might signal, is important protection against allowing serious conditions to go unchecked.

Treating the symptoms

We should take a holistic approach to treating disease and rather than treat symptoms in isolation, search for their underlying cause or causes.

For example, for an acid stomach with pain after eating you might chew antacid tablets rather than review your dietary, smoking, and drinking habits, and the level of stress in your life. The antacid tablets may relieve the symptoms, but the symptoms will likely recur unless you address the cause.

Be aware of your health

Monitoring one's health does not mean becoming a hypochondriac who sees every symptom as confirmation that he or she has terminal cancer, but rather developing an awareness of how the body functions when it is healthy. The problem is that if we run ourselves ragged, drink and smoke too much, and eat a lot of fast food, we probably never feel really well and full of vitality, so there is no yardstick to measure when we are suffering symptoms that might require medical attention.

We might become used to having frequent colds, coughs, indigestion, constipation, headaches, and low energy levels if we lead an unhealthy lifestyle, and whereas we are not exactly ill, neither are we healthy. And these minor symptoms of disease could signal the potential for more serious conditions such as chronic heart or respiratory conditions.

A yardstick for good health

Do you feel "a bit under the weather" most of the time? So many of us become accustomed to feeling below par, that we may well fail to notice symptoms that signal disease.

A yardstick against which to measure basic good health is:

- A healthy digestion; no bloating, constipation, heartburn.
- Enough energy to do what you want.
- A clear, active mind and a good memory.
- A body largely free from aches and pains.
- Good, restful sleep.

If your health does not regularly measure up to this healthy yardstick, it is time to take action.

Take a break from any energy-sapping habits, even for just a few weeks, to allow your body the chance to feel balanced and healthy. Notice how you feel when you sleep well and wake with a clear head, no hangover, no tight chest from cigarettes, no bloated stomach from too many pizzas and coffees. This is being well. Once you have experienced this feeling of well-being, the genuine symptoms of ill health will be clearer and easier to recognize.

Regular checkups

Because all the body's systems interact, any problem in one area could signal, or lead to, problems in another. This is one reason why it is so important to maintain the body in good condition, for much the same reasons as you would your car.

Prevention is better than cure so regular checkups are important. These should include: dental, eye, breast, weight, and mole or skin lesion monitoring; for women, gynecological checks, for men, prostate checks. As you get older you should have regular blood pressure monitoring, breast screening, and consider an occasional full-body screening.

Never ignore an unusual symptom, such as pain, discomfort, a lump or lesion, or persistent change in bowel habit. Never mask a new symptom by taking drugs to suppress it without first having it properly investigated by a health professional. Knowledge about the symptoms of ill health and being consciously aware of our bodies, make us better able to maintain health and energy, and to avoid disease.

infections

Infections are the most common cause of disease, and low energy is often an early symptom. In the West, we have the resources to make most infectious diseases preventable or treatable, but in underdeveloped countries they are often fatal. Resistance to infection can be greatly enhanced by maintaining a healthy immune system.

Types of infection

There are basically four types of organisms, or germs, that can cause infections: bacteria, viruses, fungi, and protozoa, and also more complex organisms, such as the intestinal worm. They can enter the body in the air we inhale, from food or drink we ingest, and through major or minor skin wounds.

The degree of damage germs can do depends on the body's resistance to infection. This is influenced by age, nutrition, and general physical and mental health – emotional trauma and an unhealthy lifestyle both weaken the immune system.

Bacteria This type of infection can occur anywhere in the body. Bacterial infections, such as pneumonia and septicemia, can be treated with antibiotics.

Viruses These commonly cause respiratory tract infections such as colds and flu. Viral infections, including measles, mumps, and HIV, cannot be treated with antibiotics; some respond to antiviral drugs; some can be prevented by immunization.

Fungi Athlete's foot is a fungal infection and can be treated with antifungal drugs.

Parasites Parasitic infections include malaria and toxoplasmosis. Treatment for these and nonprotozoan parasites such as intestinal worms is with drugs that eliminate the specific parasite.

Controlling infection

Infective organisms live all around us but good general health and hygiene will minimize the risks. Most vulnerable are the very young and very old, anyone with existing disease, and those suffering depression or emotional trauma.

Important factors in protection against infection include:

■ Good personal and environmental hygiene.

■ Good nutrition.

■ Stress reduction.

■ Immunization where appropriate.

■ Avoid crowded places where germs are plentiful.

Energy-sapping infections

Tiredness and lethargy are common symptoms of infections such as colds, flu, chronic fatigue syndrome, infectious mononucleosis, and diseases such as malaria.

Colds Over 200 different viruses cause colds. The virus spreads by droplet infection or by direct contact. It should clear within two weeks without medication.

We are surrounded by bugs, but a healthy immune system will prevent these organisms from causing serious illness.

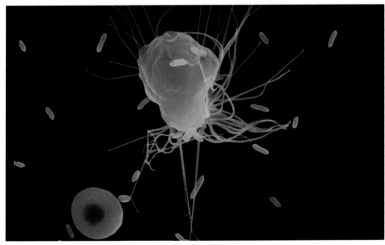

Symptoms include tiredness, runny or stuffed nose, sore throat, blocked sinuses.

Treatment Conventional treatment includes plenty of fluids, rest, and over-the-counter cold remedies. Complementary treatments include vitamin C, zinc, or homeopathy.

Influenza The many strains of the flu virus are highly infectious and spread, like colds, by droplet infection or by direct contact. Symptoms usually last for around one week. Secondary infection is a risk and flu can be serious for anyone whose immune system is compromised, such as asthmatics, diabetics, or the elderly.

Symptoms include tiredness, high fever, swollen glands, aching limbs and head, and sore throat. Depression and ongoing lethargy are later complications.

Treatment Conventional treatment includes bed rest, plenty of fluids, acetaminophen for aches, pains, and fever, and possibly an antiviral drug. Complementary treatment could include acupuncture, homeopathy, shiatsu massage, and supplements of vitamin C, echinecea and other herbs, and transfer factor.

Infectious mononucleosis This is caused by the Epstein-Barr virus (EBV), one of the herpes group. It is transmitted mainly by direct contact – it is often known as the "kissing disease" – but also by droplet infection. The virus has a four- to six-week incubation period, but can be carried without ever developing symptoms. Diagnosis is by blood test or throat swab.

Symptoms include swollen glands in the neck, underarms, and groin, fever, sore throat, and extreme tiredness, which can persist for many months. Symptoms, except tiredness, disappear within about two weeks.

PNEUMONIA

This is infection of the air sacs (alveoli) in the lungs, usually from a bacteria infection. Legionnaire's disease is one form. Symptoms usually appear rapidly, within a few hours, and include high fever, cough, shortness of breath, chest pain that is worse when you breathe in. Seek medical help immediately if you have these symptoms.

Treatment Conventional treatment includes bed rest, fluids and medication to relieve symptoms. Complementary treatment is with large doses of vitamin C.

Chronic fatigue syndrome (CFS) Complex and poorly understood by most conventional M.D.s, this multisystem disease is associated with symptoms in the back, endocrine glands, brain, muscles, immune system, and may affect blod coagulation. It has been associated with infections, heavy metal and other environmental toxins, and injuries, especially of the neck and back. The fatigue and mental fog can be very debilitating and treatment by specialized experts is essential.

Symptoms include extreme fatigue for six months or more, plus muscle or joint pain, headache, poor concentration, sleep disturbance – all made worse by exercise.

Treatment Conventional medicine treats symptoms with painkillers or antidepressants; sufferers are encouraged to manage symptoms with stress reduction, light exercise, physiotherapy, diet, and social support. Complementary treatment includes cognitive therapy, herbal medicine, vitamin B12 supplements, acupuncture, and homeopathy.

Malaria The world's most common parasitic infection is responsible for 10 million infections and two million deaths – mostly children – every year. It is spread by malaria-infected mosquitoes when they bite. Seek advice from your doctor about precautions before visiting a malarial zone.

Symptoms include tiredness, fever, vomiting, muscle pains, and headache.

Treatment Antimalarial prescription drugs. (See p. 79.)

Intestinal worms Threadworm infestation is usually caused by eating worm eggs in contaminated food or from pets. The eggs then hatch in the intestines. Tapeworms are contracted by eating poorly cooked pork, beef, and raw fish. There may be no symptoms and diagnosis is made when eggs, worms, or portions of worms are found in the feces.

Symptoms include tiredness because essential nutrients are being consumed by the parasites, increased appetite, diarrhea, severe anal itching.

Treatment Conventional treatment uses anthelmintic drugs and advice about avoiding reinfection. Complementary treatment includes herbal medicine.

chronic
diseases

Chronic, or long-term disease is debilitating not only because of the physical symptoms but also because you have to reeducate yourself about how to live your life, learning to be realistic about how much energy you have to achieve what you want. But energy levels, even in chronic disease, can be improved with diet and good management.

Take control of your disease

Whatever the disease, it is important to take an integrated approach to its management. Medical treatment should be augmented by complementary therapies where appropriate, and the impact of symptoms can be minimized with a healthy diet and an appropriate exercise program. Taking control of disease is good for your mental health, too. If you are suffering chronic ill health the following advice will help you feel better:

■ Find out everything you can about your illness; talk to your doctor, read journals, and use the Internet to keep abreast of advances in treatment.

■ Talk to fellow sufferers for support and information about management.

■ Make sure your general health is as good as it can be.

■ Be realistic about your energy levels and do not tire yourself out.

■ Think positively; when it comes to healing and the immune system, the mind-body connection is very strong.

■ Take a holistic, integrated approach; use conventional medicine and complementary therapies in combination whenever appropriate.

Do not feel that because you are suffering from a chronic condition you cannot take advantage of the dietary, exercise, and complementary health options described in this book.

When tiredness means trouble

Lack of energy is often one of the first symptoms of the following chronic conditions, but tiredness does not necessarily mean serious illness. As a general rule of thumb, unexplained tiredness that persists and is accompanied by some of the other symptoms listed below may signal illness and you should consult your doctor.

Anemia There are many different causes for this, a blood disorder where hemoglobin, the oxygen-carrying component in red blood cells, is deficient. The most common is iron deficiency that can result from excessive blood loss due to a heavy period, a major injury, a bleeding ulcer, poor diet, pregnancy, and less commonly from malabsorption in the intestine.
Symptoms include tiredness, pallor, faintness, and shortness of breath on exercise.
Treatment Conventional treatment includes iron supplements, plus dietary advice. Complementary treatment may include vitamin C to aid iron absorption.

Cancer Broadly, this is when cells mutate and multiply inappropriately. Cancer can be caused by factors including: genetic, nutritional, age, and environmental agents such as tobacco smoke, asbestos, chemicals, sunlight, and radiation. But the most common causes of all adult cancers are smoking, sunlight, and a poor diet high in saturated fat, alcohol, and food-chain chemicals.
Symptoms include unexplained tiredness and/or weight loss, which are common to most cancers. Specific symptoms vary depending on the type of cancer; for example, a breast lump may indicate breast cancer, or a change in bowel habits and rectal bleeding may indicate colon cancer.

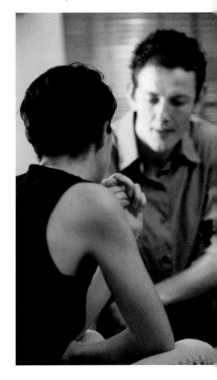

Even if you are suffering from a chronic disease, you can still do lots to raise your energy levels.

Treatment Conventional treatment can include surgery, radiotherapy, chemotherapy, and counseling. Complementary treatment may include nutritional supplements, high-dose antioxidant therapy, herbal medicine, visualization, acupuncture, and relaxation techniques.

Prevention is better than cure, and it makes sense to take preventive measures against cancer where possible. Don't smoke, do eat a balanced diet, maintain a healthy immune system, and ensure you are on preventive screening programs.

Hepatitis Chronic hepatitis is when the liver has been inflamed for at least six months. It has a number of causes, including viral infection from hepatitis C, and occasionally B and D, alcohol or drug abuse, and an autoimmune response, where the immune system attacks the liver itself. The condition puts the sufferer at increased risk of cirrhosis and cancer of the liver.

Symptoms include tiredness, loss of appetite or vomiting, yellowing of the skin and whites of the eyes, and a swollen or aching abdomen, although the disease is sometimes symptom free in the early stages.

Treatment Depending on the cause and severity of the hepatitis, conventional treatment includes antiviral, steroid, or immunosuppressant drugs. Complementary treatment includes homeopathy, nutrition therapy, and dietary supplements.

Human immunodeficiency virus (HIV) This virus weakens the body's ability to resist infections and cancer. Having HIV does not mean carriers will necessarily contract acquired immunodeficiency syndrome (AIDS), although it is thought to be one of the causes.

It is possible to harbor the virus for many years without showing any symptoms, or to succumb quickly to infection. Transmission occurs through direct contact with body fluids, mainly blood, semen, and breast milk. Prevention includes avoiding unprotected sex or contaminated injection needles.

Early general symptoms include tiredness, fever, swollen lymph glands, sore throat, and a rash. Specific symptoms vary from person to person.

Treatment Conventional treatment uses antiretroviral and antibiotic drugs alongside medication and counseling to treat symptoms. Complementary treatments include nutritional therapy, herbal medicine, acupuncture, aromatherapy, and massage.

Irritable bowel syndrome (IBS) This describes a collection of symptoms that tend to flare up with varying degrees of frequency and severity over long periods of time, sometimes years. It is thought by some to be triggered by food intolerance, particularly yeast sensitivity, to be stress related, and to have a strong psychological component. It often follows bacterial infections in the bowel.

Symptoms include bloating, abdominal pain, wind, diarrhea or constipation, nausea, sometimes mucus in the feces, and tiredness.

Treatment Conventional treatment includes diet, antispasmodic drugs for abdominal or intestinal pain, and remedies for diarrhea and constipation. Complementary treatment includes relaxation techniques, nutritional advice including eliminating food sensitivities, shiatsu massage, yoga, herbal supplements, and homeopathy.

Lyme disease Although up until recently this has been a disease contracted mostly in North America, it is now more common in British woods and parkland where there are deer. A bacterial infection, it is transmitted by a bite from a deer tick. Lyme disease is not usually dangerous if treated promptly but left untreated the parasite can attack organs such as the heart, and the central nervous system, resulting in chronic health problems.

Symptoms include a "bull's-eye" rash around the bite, tiredness, fever, and flulike symptoms of headache, stiff neck, and painful joints, which usually come on two to four weeks after being bitten.

Treatment Conventional treatment is mainly antibiotics, with NSAIDs for joint pain. There is an immunization if you are particularly at risk. Complementary treatment, in conjunction with antibiotics, includes homeopathic and herbal remedies.

CHECK YOUR FECES

Streaks of fresh blood in your feces, if the amounts are small, are most probably due to hemorrhoids. But if the amount of blood is larger it could make your stool look almost black. If you have persistent rectal bleeding, difficulty or pain having a normal bowel movement, or are aware of a lump in that area, it is important to consult your doctor, as these may be signs of colon cancer.

allergy and food intolerance

A growing proportion of the population suffers from life-threatening allergies. Many lives are blighted by mild but persistent reactions to a variety of allergens. Other people, although not allergic, have a sensitivity to certain foods. Both allergies and sensitivities can drastically impair energy.

The antibody response

The body's immune system is a very sophisticated, protective mechanism against infection and disease. First, any germ has to break into the body, invading the protective skin and mucus-lined passages, which help to trap and expel organisms. Then it has to negotiate the inflammatory response where it is doused with chemicals designed to destroy it. And if it evades these two barriers, then, depending on the nature of the germ, it comes up against two further immune responses, the cellular and the antibody response. These reactions to invading organisms is going on in our bodies all the time.

What is an allergic reaction?

When the antibody response has gotten out of balance and the body overreacts to a substance that should be harmless, such as pollen, this is an allergic reaction. The first time the substance, known as an allergen, is ingested the body becomes sensitized but there is no obvious reaction. Subsequently, when the substance comes into contact with the body, histamine is released, which triggers inflammation.

Some allergic reactions are immediate and life threatening (see box opposite); others develop gradually over a few hours, sometimes a few days, with symptoms ranging from mild to very severe. Rarely, there can be long-term organ damage.

Allergy symptoms Common allergic symptoms vary, depending on which area of the body is affected, but all the reactions take the form of inflammation. For example, in allergic rhinitis, known as hay fever if it occurs seasonally, the symptoms are watery, itchy, swollen eyes, an itchy, runny nose, sneezing, fatigue, and headache.

Foods, drugs, or insect stings Symptoms include swelling of the lips, face, and throat, nausea and vomiting, wheezing, and an itchy red rash anywhere on the body; often the rash is raised or has white bumps. This is called urticaria or hives.
Treatment Conventional treatment includes avoidance of the allergen, over-the-counter oral antihistamines, or the topical application of calamine lotion. Complementary treatments such as herbal medicine, acupuncture, or hypnotherapy may help but conventional medical advice should be sought for severe allergic reactions.

Who gets allergies?

Everyone is exposed to pollen, house dust, and pet hair, but some people have an allergic response where others do not. Research has not yet pinpointed what gives a person what is known as an "atopic" disposition – an inherent predisposition to

ANAPHYLACTIC SHOCK

An allergic response can occasionally be extreme, immediate, and potentially fatal. This is called anaphylaxis and thankfully is rare. It is most commonly caused by beestings, foods including nuts, fish, and strawberries, or an adverse reaction to certain drugs such as penicillin.

Once you have experienced anaphylactic shock with a particular substance, avoid that substance and carry a syringe containing adrenalin with you at all times, which you, or someone with you, can inject immediately if you suffer the adverse reaction. You should also consider wearing a bracelet or carrying a card to inform others in an emergency. Symptoms include: hives, difficulty breathing, swollen face, lips, and tongue, flushing, diarrhea, and shock. Emergency hospital treatment is required for this condition.

allergies – which makes them vulnerable to common allergens such as pollen, and animal fur that may cause asthma and eczema.

A genetic factor, childhood infection, pollution, "leaky gut syndrome," stress, and psychological factors are all thought to be potential triggers. Even childhood immunizations are thought by some to increase vunerability to allergies. Whatever the cause, in the last 15 years asthma cases have increased, with children particularly affected. However, having a healthy immune system greatly increases your chances of minimizing the discomfort of all allergic reactions.

Allergy testing

Tests can help pinpoint the cause of many persistent allergic reactions. These include:

■ **Skin test** Dilute amounts of potential allergens are pricked into the skin.

■ **Blood test** This involves a biochemical technique that checks for specific antibodies known as IgG antibodies, thought to be present in allergic reactions. Two techniques are used: ELISA (enzyme-linked immunosorbent assay) and RAST (radioallergosorbent test).

Some allergy testing techniques such as Electromagnetic testing, hair analysis, and applied kinesiology are more controversial and not accepted in mainstream medicine, but there is some evidence that these techniques do work.

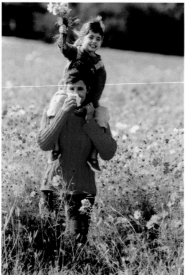

■ **Electromagnetic testing** It involves attaching the patient to a computer that measures the electrical vibrations that flow through the body's acupuncture points in response to potential allergens.

Allergic reactions seem to be on the increase, with children particularly affected.

■ **Hair analysis** This measures the reaction when possible allergens are combined with compounds eliminated in strands of hair.

■ **Applied kinesiology** Here, sensitivity to foodstuffs or allergens is assessed by testing a person's muscle strength while in close proximity to a substance. The diagnosis is based on the theory that energy flow through the body, which is affected by allergens, is reflected in muscle strength.

Avoiding allergens

Once you have identified the substance to which you are allergic, the next problem is avoiding it. It might seem simple, for instance, not to eat peanuts, but many processed foods, and foods bought in shops, restaurants, and takeout stores are contaminated in the manufacturing, marketing, or cooking process, or contain unexpected ingredients such as peanut oil. So, it is important to be vigilant about everything you consume; read food ingredient and additive labels, and ask about ingredients in restaurants.

Airborne allergens such as pollen, house dust, and pet hairs are equally hard to avoid because obviously we must all breathe.

Various measures can help:

■ Stay indoors when the pollen count is high, particularly mornings, evenings, and when there is freshly mown grass around. Use an air filter indoors.

■ Replace pillows and quilts with synthetic fiber filling, cover mattresses with plastic, replace carpets with wood floors; clean and dust the house regularly.

■ Avoid keeping pets, or spending too much time in houses with pets.

■ Drink plenty of plain water to dilute the allergen and clear the system.

Food intolerance

Food intolerance is not the same as an allergic reaction where there is a specific, measurable immune response in the body; rather it is more an oversensitivity to a particular food or group of foods.

It is thought by some experts to be extremely prevalent and largely responsible for the tiredness and low energy so many of us complain about these days. If you think you have a food intolerance it is best to consult a qualified nutritionist, naturopath, or kinesiologist, who will supervise testing with techniques mentioned above, and advise on treatment.

Symptoms of food intolerance These vary, but the general symptoms include: tiredness, bloating, excessive gas, lethargy (particularly after eating), erratic bowel habits, tendency to allergies, and skin irritations.

Foods most commonly thought to promote sensitivity are:

■ **Gluten** Found predominantly in wheat but in smaller amounts in rye, oats, and barley. Wheat is responsible for the malabsorption syndrome known as celiac disease.

■ **Milk** Milk proteins, lactose – the sugar found in milk and dairy products – and the chemicals produced when milk is treated, are all considered culprits.

Other substances that do not cause actual food intolerances, but that have been pinpointed by a growing number of nutritionists as being associated with low energy levels in some people, are refined sugar, products that contain yeast, such as alcohol and bread (see page 69), and the nitrates found in many additives and preservatives in processed food and meat. The jury is still out on genetically modified food, but many scientists and nutritionists are worried that not enough research has been done into the safety of these foods.

What causes food intolerance

Food intolerances cannot always be blamed only on the causative agent. They are also thought to stem from digestive problems such as low stomach acid, lack of digestive enzymes, or agents that inflame the bowel and disturb the natural balance of healthy bacteria in the intestine, leading to a defective absorption of nutrients known as "leaky intestinal syndrome" and overgrowth of yeast and other dangerous bacteria.

Leaky intestinal syndrome The small intestine is where the nutrients from digested food are absorbed into the bloodstream. A healthy intestine is very selective and allows only the smallest nutrient molecules through. But if the intestinal wall is damaged, larger molecules, including whole bacteria and toxins, escape and are absorbed into the blood, which may provoke an adverse response resulting in the symptoms of food sensitivity and allergic reactions such as skin rashes.

Many agents can cause the breakdown of the intestinal wall, including infections, antibiotics, and NSAIDs, and the abuse of the digestive system by the usual suspects: stress, poor diet, smoking, alcohol, and environmental chemicals.

Chronic leaky gut has been implicated in conditions such as asthma, inflammatory bowel disease, rheumatoid arthritis, and multiple sclerosis.

Symptoms In addition to the general symptoms of food intolerance (see p. 68), these include sensitivity to wheat and dairy products.

Treatment Conventional medicine does not recognize this syndrome despite extensive data. Complementary therapy includes diagnosis with a laboratory test called a "intestinal permeability test," then treats with diet, herbal medicine, and supplements. This is best supervised by a qualified nutritionist.

Yeast overgrowth Yeast products such as bread, alcohol, vinegar, and matured cheese have been taken for centuries with no adverse reaction. So why suddenly is yeast such a villain in digestive health?

Antibiotics, especially if taken long term, are the most common culprits. They kill harmful bacteria but they also kill healthy bacteria, which are fundamental to the digestion and other body processes.

This absence of bacteria also gives the opportunity for fungi such as the yeast organism, *Candida albicans*, to flourish. This overgrowth of yeast – especially if it is encouraged by yeast-containing foods and foods such as sugar that are thought to promote yeast growth – contributes to food sensitivity and poor absorption of nutrients.

Symptoms In addition to the general symptoms of food intolerance (see p. 68), there may be frequent oral and vaginal thrush infections and cystitis.

Treatment Conventional medication for infection. Complementary treatment includes probiotic supplements, and nutritional support for the intestinal tract.

To help prevent digestive problems if you are taking antibiotics you should consider also taking probiotics – such as *Lactobacillus acidophilus* – to replace the healthy intestinal flora. (See p. 89.)

Elimination diets

We discuss various diets to improve energy in the "Options" section, but a favorite way of pinpointing a food intolerance is by eliminating all the most likely foods from your diet, such as wheat, dairy products, foods you crave, and foods you suspect, for two weeks. If you have a food sensitivity, you will probably feel better after two weeks and can start replacing foods one at a time to see if they cause an adverse reaction. This process should not be undertaken without medical supervision.

hormonal
imbalances

Because hormones affect all the body systems, if their levels of production are thrown out of balance energy levels are disrupted. Normal hormone production does fluctuate in response to a variety of factors. But sometimes one of the hormone-secreting glands malfunctions and it is important to be able to recognize the difference between normal fluctuations and disease.

Hormone imbalance and low energy

Hormones are chemicals that are secreted from different sites throughout the body. Some are secreted by specific hormone-producing glands, such as the thyroid and adrenal gland, some are manufactured in cells within organs, such as the kidneys and pancreas. Hormone release is regulated by the part of the brain known as the hypothalamus. Hormones send messages around the body via the bloodstream that stimulate a range of different body functions, often in a chain reaction through the system. Hormone imbalances in particular are connected with mood swings, tiredness, and lethargy, and more commonly affect women than men.

Hypothyroidism Thyroid hormones (including thyroxine) are essential for metabolism – temperature control and how we burn fuel – nervous system function, and also sexual function. The thyroid gland can malfunction on two levels; over production of the thyroid hormones (hyperthyroidism), or underproduction (hypothyroidism) where symptoms reflect a slowing down of the metabolism.

   The causes for hypothyroidism are numerous and include:
■ **Thyroiditis**, an inflammation of the thyroid gland. It can be due to viral infection,

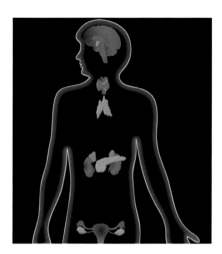

or an auto-immune disorder called Hashimoto's disease, most common in middle-aged women, where antibodies attack the thyroid gland.

Thyroiditis can affect women after giving birth, although this form usually resolves without treatment.

■ **Iodine deficiency** due to malabsorption of iodine as a result of a damaged thyroid gland or from a diet low in iodine-rich seafood – no longer common in the West.

■ **Drugs** such as lithium and those used to treat epilepsy.

■ **Stress** because cortisol, the stress hormone, can suppress thyroxine production.

Energy levels may be disrupted by fluctuating hormone levels, which can have many different causes.

■ **Pollutants** such as mercury and lead may inhibit thyroxine production.

■ **Lack of thyroid secreting hormone (TSH)** when the pituitary gland fails to secrete enough TSH to maintain levels of thyroid hormones. This happens only rarely.

Symptoms Hypothyroidism causes a generalized slowing down of body functions giving rise to extreme tiredness, weight gain, slow heart rate and speech, depression, sensitivity to cold, fluid retention, constipation, dry and coarse skin, and hair loss; also goiter, a swelling in the front of the neck due to thyroid gland enlargement.

These symptoms may develop slowly over weeks or months, and hypothyroidism is sometimes difficult to diagnose because of the often insidious onset. If you experience three or more symptoms over a sustained period of time you should seek medical advice.

Treatment Conventional treatment includes thyroid hormone (thyroxine) replacement, or nutritional supplements of iodine. Complementary alternatives include nutritional therapy, acupuncture, yoga, and relaxation techniques.

Adrenal gland disorders "Adrenal insufficiency" is thought by some to be a common cause of tiredness and low energy levels, but many doctors do not recognize this as a valid condition.

Adrenal insufficiency has no identifiable cause but it is thought to affect people with persistently high levels of stress hormones, which build up and put a strain on all the organs, leading to chemical imbalance and adrenal insufficiency.

Symptoms These include tiredness not helped by sleep, low energy reserves, feeling exhausted by exercise, low blood pressure, dizziness on standing, and irritability if meals are not regular.

Treatment Complementary treatment includes herbal and nutritional supplements, cortisol supplements, and stress management. If you think you may suffer from adrenal insufficiency you could consult a qualified naturopath or a doctor who practices integrated medicine – one who uses conventional and complementary treatments.

Hormones and low energy in women

A woman's reproductive system is governed by hormones and most women experience the effects of hormonal disruption at some stage in their lives, whether it be during menstruation, pregnancy, menopause, or because of a medical problem such as endometriosis. Tiredness and lack of energy are the most common symptoms of which women complain when there is hormonal imbalance.

Premenstrual syndrome (PMS) This is caused by imbalances in the circulating levels of sex hormones, estrogen and progesterone, in the days before menstruation. PMS is thought to be made worse by a combination of factors, many not clearly understood, such as vitamin and mineral deficiencies, stress, and a diet containing too much chocolate and caffeine.

Symptoms It is said that at least one third of all women experience symptoms, though they vary in type and severity. These include tiredness, irritability, anxiety, mood swings that are sometimes violent, tearfulness, bloating, breast tenderness, headaches, and food cravings – for sugar or chocolate in particular.

Treatment Conventional treatment includes managing the symptoms, for example with painkillers and sometimes the oral contraceptive pill. Complementary treatment includes diet, osteopathy, reflexology, meditation, and natural progesterone. It is worth consulting a complementary practitioner if your symptoms disrupt your life.

Menorrhagia Heavy menstrual bleeding is one of the most common causes of fatigue, and it can result in iron deficiency anemia. The cause is not always apparent but can be due to problems within the uterus such as fibroids, polyps, endometriosis, or endometrial cancer.

Other causes include hypothyroidism, sustained stress, and the use of an intra-uterine contraceptive device (IUD).

Symptoms Heavy menstrual bleeding for more than seven days with noticeable clots in the blood, tiredness, and lower abdominal pain.

Treatment Conventional treatment may include measuring hormone levels, an ultrasound scan and a hysteroscopy to examine the uterus, surgical removal of any uterine growth, and iron supplements to combat anemia. Complementary treatment includes stress management, massage, yoga, and nutritional supplements.

Endometriosis This is when the endometrium, which lines the uterus, grows into areas of the pelvis; on the outside of the uterus, for example, or into the fallopian tubes, ovaries, bowel, or bladder. The cause is not known.

Symptoms Intense lower abdominal pain, particularly before menstruation, irregular and sometimes heavy periods, and pain on sexual intercourse.

Treatment Conventional treatment may include the combined oral contraceptive pill to block the menstrual cycle, surgical removal of parts of the endometrium, or, sometimes, hysterectomy. Hormone studies may be helpful.

Menopause The natural end of a woman's menstrual cycle is characterized by a drop in estrogen production and a cessation of progesterone production. For most women it causes few problems but for some the symptoms are severe and ongoing.

Symptoms These include hot flashes, tiredness, mood swings, anxiety, tearfulness, interrupted sleep, night sweats, fat deposits around the stomach, and vaginal dryness.

Treatment Conventional treatment includes hormone replacement therapy (HRT). Complementary treatment includes natural hormones, diet, and meditation.

depression

Tiredness and lethargy are often the first symptoms of depression. There are many different forms of the illness and even now no one really knows why some people are more susceptible to it and others not. But knowing the symptoms and available treatments will help if you think your low energy has a root in depressive illness.

What is depression?

The term "depression" covers a wide range of symptoms, which vary from person to person. Depression is usually divided into mild, moderate, and severe, diagnosed on the basis of the number and severity of symptoms present. Some forms, such as seasonal affective disorder (SAD) and postnatal depression, relate to specific events.

What makes us depressed?

The definitive cause of depressive illness is unknown but there is consensus on some of the contributing causes that fall broadly into three groups:

Biological causes Alteration in levels of proteins and amino acids essential to produce the mood enhancer, serotonin, some physical illnesses, and genetic inheritance.

Psychological causes Those prone to depression tend to think of themselves negatively, as worthless and unlovable. Other causes include lack of a healthy, loving attachment to the mother figure, or the loss of a parent in childhood.

Social causes A stressful lifestyle, poverty, emotional trauma such as bereavement or divorce, or any dramatic life change to which we find it difficult to adjust.

Diagnosing depression

The diagnosis of depression can be confused by other illnesses that mimic depressive symptoms but a persistent low mood combined with five or more of the following symptoms, which persist for two weeks or more, indicates depression.

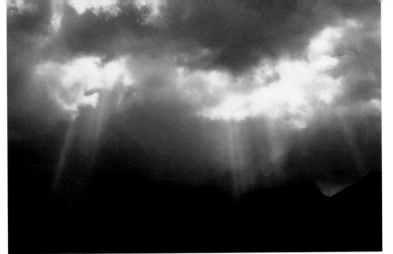

Anyone suffering a depressive episode will have low energy levels.

Symptoms Lack of energy and feeling tired all the time, ongoing low mood, loss of self-esteem and confidence, anxiety attacks, change in eating habits, disturbed sleep – particularly waking early in the morning – difficulty in concentrating and making decisions, irritability and impatience, lack of pleasure or anticipation in things you normally enjoy, loss of libido, persistent negative thoughts, self-criticism, and self-destructive behavior often manifested in thoughts of suicide.

Treatment Conventional treatment includes antidepressant drugs, such as selective serotonin re-uptake inhibitors (SSRIs), which include Prozac and Paxil, and psychological therapies. Complementary treatment includes meditation, visualization, yoga, hypnotherapy, and herbal remedies such as St. John's Wort.

Seasonal affective disorder (SAD) The production of the hormones melatonin and serotonin are affected by the reduced light during the short winter days, but it is not known why only some people are affected.

Symptoms Persistent lethargy and depression during winter that recedes as daylight hours lengthen.

Treatment All treatment includes full-spectrum light therapy to replace daylight.

Seek help Depression is an illness like any other. If your lack of energy is accompanied by some of the other symptoms discussed here, do seek help; so much can be done to alleviate depression.

adverse
reactions
to prescription
medicines

Prescription medicines can be very successful in alleviating a health problem, but because all medicines taken into the body affect the whole system, it is possible you may suffer unwanted reactions to some of these drugs.

Know your medicine

We don't take enough responsibility for the medicines we are prescribed; we tend to leave it all up to the doctor. But drugs should be taken with great care; it is your body receiving the drug and perhaps suffering its side effects, and you are the one who will be the first to realize when something is going wrong. It is vital to understand the type of drug you are taking, to know what effect it is supposed to have on your symptoms, and how soon you can expect to see or feel a difference; you must be clear about the potential side effects, both long and short term.

It is difficult sometimes to make enough time to ask the doctor all these questions in a hurried consultation, but it is always possible to talk to a pharmacist at more length, to read the information sheet that is supplied with the drug, or check out the drug's history and track record yourself on the Internet.

Drugs: precautionary measures

Before taking any drugs, you should certainly tell your doctor if you are on any other drugs, including complementary remedies. Many drugs interact badly. You should also:

■ Tell your doctor if you or a close family member have ever experienced a severe reaction to a drug.

■ Tell your doctor if you are, or might be, pregnant.

■ Find out why you are taking a drug and how long you should take it for.

■ Take the drug according to instructions from your doctor or pharmacist, and always complete the course of treatment, unless you experience a reaction.

■ Never stop taking a prescribed drug suddenly without consulting your doctor.

■ Check and make sure you understand all the drug's potential side effects.

■ Over-the-counter (OTC) medicines can be powerful so check with the pharmacist before taking any drug, and don't take unnecessary medicines.

■ If you experience an adverse reaction to any drug, seek advice from a doctor or pharmacist. If the symptoms are severe, seek urgent medical help.

Drugs to be wary of

The following commonly prescribed drugs need to be treated with particular care. They include antibiotics, antihypertensives, and antidepressants; also hormone replacement therapy and antimalarial drugs.

OVER-THE-COUNTER DRUGS

Never give aspirin to a child under the age of 12 as this might trigger a rare disease called Reye's syndrome, which causes inflammation of the brain and liver, and can be fatal. Symptoms include vomiting, drowsiness, and seizures. Check OTC cold and flu remedies for aspirin content and get urgent medical help if your child develops the above symptoms. Avoid taking aspirin or ibuprofen if you have asthma or a stomach ulcer. Use acetaminophen-based drugs as an alternative for short-term treatment.

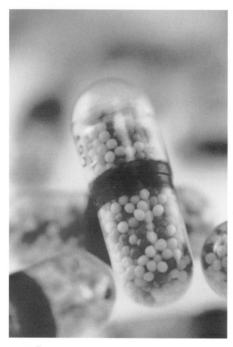

Antibiotics are over-prescribed, so make sure you really need them and take probiotics as well.

Antibiotics These are safe and effective for bacterial infections but are over-prescribed. Injudicious use can create resistant strains of bacteria, making infections more difficult to treat. Antibiotics can destroy "friendly" intestinal bacteria that can trigger yeast overgrowth (candidiasis), and cause digestive problems. (See "Food Intolerances," p. 67.)

Penicillin can cause reactions from a mild rash to a serious allergic reaction. (See "Anaphylactic shock," p. 65.)

Tetracyclines are powerful antibiotics that can inhibit bone and tooth development, and occasionally cause kidney damage, and therefore they tend not to be prescribed to children or pregnant women.

If you are prescribed antibiotics, ask your doctor if they are really necessary, and if you do take them, then take probiotic supplements as well.

Antihypertensives These treat high blood pressure. There are various ones that lower the blood pressure in different ways and they include:

ACE inhibitors, alpha- and beta-blockers, diuretics There are many possible side effects from these drugs but one distressing reaction with some antihypertensives is male impotence. The problem usually goes away when the medication is stopped so your doctor may suggest an alternative drug. Never stop taking an antihypertensive without first seeking medical advice. Sudden withdrawal can cause blood pressure to rise dangerously, increasing the risk of stroke and heart attack.

Antidepressants Selective serotonin re-uptake inhibitors (SSRIs), such as Prozac and Paxil, are currently the most popular drug treatment for depressive symptoms, and have fewer side effects than many other antidepressant drugs. But they have had some very bad press concerning adverse reactions in a minority of users who develop suicidal tendencies, high anxiety, and aggression (sometimes murderous), often within a few days of starting to take the drug.

However, SSRIs are very successful in alleviating depressive symptoms, and the main side effect for most people is loss of libido and ability to achieve orgasm.

Combine antidepressant drug therapy with complementary therapies wherever possible, and be alert to any sudden changes in mood in those taking SSRIs.

Antimalarials Mefloquine (Lariam), is used prophylactically – i.e., to prevent rather than cure – against malaria. Recent claims state that it can cause severe psychosis, with paranoia, mood swings, suicide, and thoughts of suicide in a minority of people.

Malaria is a serious disease and it is important to protect against it, not least by preventing mosquito bites where possible. If you are traveling to a malarial area, either begin taking Lariam at least three weeks before traveling to allow time to notice any adverse reaction, or try one of the newer antimalarial drugs.

Hormone replacement therapy (HRT) Menopause is a normal life process, not a disease. HRT is taken by menopausal women to alleviate the uncomfortable symptoms of estrogen withdrawal: hot flashes, night sweats, and mood swings.

Only a minority of women taking HRT, those with at least five menopausal symptoms (see p. 73), benefit from it; the rest would be better using natural remedies such as diet, exercise, and supplements.

HRT is no longer a first-line treatment for the symptoms of menopause. It has been shown to increase the risk of heart attacks, strokes, blood clots, and brest cancer.

Physicians are beginning to turn to diet, exercise, and certain supplements and herbs to treat symptoms of menopause: vitamin E, vitamin C, and black cohosh are frequent choices.

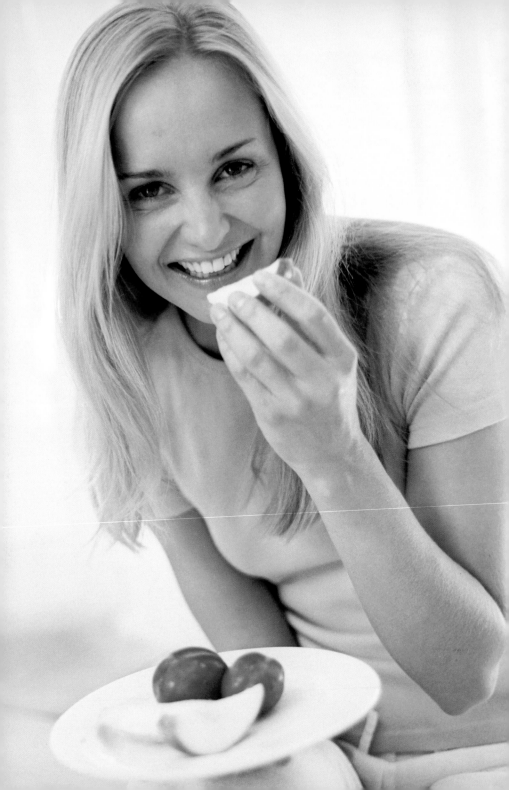

all the
options

We are all different, and there are many diets, exercise ideas, and supportive complementary therapies to help each of us start our personal energizing program.

Take your time to find the right one for you, and don't think of it as a quick fix. What you want is a health and energy plan for life that is flexible, manageable, and above all, enjoyable.

lifestyle changes

Changing the way we live is never easy. To achieve
higher energy levels, we must go the extra mile and
change our comfortable, but unhealthy, habits. You
are probably starting to understand how you may be
sabotaging your energy levels and already beginning
to modify your lifestyle.

To support this goal, the second half of the book
offers tricks and techniques to help eliminate the
energy-depleting elements in your life. But this is not
the whole story. We also outline lots of ideas for diet,
exercise, and relaxation, which you can put in place
of those bad habits. And we tell you about the
various complementary therapies that can support you
in your quest to boost your energy.

There is nothing painful or too extreme, so have fun.

diet

The way we eat is the single most important element in the quest for high energy. Exercise, relaxation, and positive emotions are vital, too, but without a healthy diet we stand absolutely no chance of achieving healthy energy levels. Good nutrition is not only about the food we have, but also about how we buy, store, cook, and eat it. Good nutrition encompasses our whole attitude to food, and the amount and quality of water we drink. In this section we discuss detoxing, a balanced diet, supplements, and juicing.

Healthy eating for energy

The word "diet" strikes fear into many hearts these days. We have come to see food as forbidden fruit. The more we diet and obsess about food, the fatter we get, because we are throwing our digestive processes into disarray with all the inconsistencies of low this, high that, lots of one thing, none of another, as is so often recommended by many modern-day diets. We may also disrupt our energy levels.

Eat for health and energy, not for weight loss, and not only will you lose weight, but you will also look fantastic. Changing your eating habits for the better allows your palette to adjust without too much effort; the more you eat good, healthy food, the more you want to. And don't beat yourself up about lapses, just start to introduce your body to a healthier eating plan and you will love the difference it makes.

Detox

Although conventional medicine still brackets body-detoxing with alternative medical practice, before embarking on a new energy eating plan, many nutritionists now suggest cleansing your system first. Detoxing gives your body a real energy boost, and you'll have clearer skin, brighter eyes, and a calmer mind.

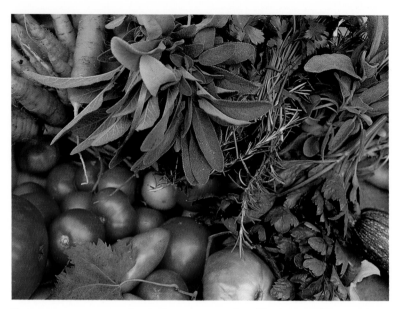

To improve your energy levels, boost your intake of fresh vegetables and fruit.

There are many different detoxification diets; the most extreme is a water fast where you eat nothing and drink only water for 24 hours. If you have never fasted before it would be wiser to start with a more moderate plan that includes fruit and fruit juice over 24 hours, or with a week eating only rice and vegetables. Only attempt a water fast or a juice-only detox if you can rest at home for the day.

If you are ill, on medication, pregnant, or breast-feeding, then fasting is not advisable, except perhaps under professional guidance.

During a fast, avoid strenuous exercise and keep warm. You might feel light-headed, irritable, nauseated, or headachey; these are effects of the body eliminating toxins. If you feel ill, stop fasting. On the day before and for a few days after fasting, eat lightly and avoid stimulants or food such as red meat or processed food.

Detoxification is aided by colonic irrigation (see p. 125), saunas, steam baths, and skinbrushing, but when fasting try these only under professional supervision.

24-hour fruit juice detox Make a huge fresh fruit salad of papaya, banana, pear or apple, grapes, plums, peaches, nectarines, and berries such as raspberries, strawberries, and cherries. Mix with unsweetened fruit juice. Eat a medium portion for breakfast, lunch, and dinner. In between the salad meals drink lots of plain mineral or filtered water, and any herbal tea of your choice (see p. 95–97).

One week rice and vegetable fast Eat only raw and steamed, preferably organic, vegetables and brown rice for a week. Between meals drink only plain mineral or filtered water and herbal tea.

Water

We have discussed the importance of drinking water to flush toxins through our system (see p. 29), but how much water should we drink? Most nutrition experts suggest between 1.5–2 quarts (1.5–2 liters) of water (ideally mineral or filtered) a day. This may sound like a lot but it is vital for energy, concentration, the digestive system, and for our general mood; we become irritable when we are thirsty and dehydrated.

Drinking a lot while eating a meal dilutes digestive enzymes; it is best to carry a bottle of fresh mineral or filtered water and drink little and often throughout the day, between meals, starting when you wake in the morning. Keep fizzy mineral water to a minimum; it contains carbon dioxide and the bubbles can make your stomach feel "gassy." Replace coffee and tea with herbal infusions, or a mug of hot water.

Energy foods

Energy foods fall principally into three groups: fruit and vegetables; grains, nuts, and seeds; and proteins.

Fruit and vegetables One thing we can do to boost energy levels and our immune system more than any other is make sure that fruit and vegetables comprise at least 50 percent of our daily diet. In many homes the average daily diet includes no more than one or two portions. Fruit and vegetables are high in fiber, low in fat, and rich in vitamins, minerals, and phytochemicals that boost the immune system.

Raw versus cooked The principle of a raw food diet is that vital nutrients are not lost through cooking, and the digestive enzymes released as we chew it kick-start the digestive process. This is said to make raw food very high in nutritional energy. However, raw food is better for you only if it is being properly digested, and for the elderly, or people with digestive problems, a diet containing a lot of raw food can be difficult to tolerate, and may cause diarrhea and gas. A good balance would be 50 percent raw to 50 percent lightly steamed or stir fried.

High-energy fruit and vegetables include: apples, apricots, dried figs, red and purple berries, beets, cabbage, broccoli, watercress, spinach, celery, carrots, avocados, parsley, and olive oil.

Grains, nuts, and seeds Cereal grains are usually seen as carbohydrates but for most of the world wholegrain is the chief source of protein and energy. Refined grains are mainly carbohydrate and can affect blood sugar imbalance because they release sugar too quickly into the bloodstream (see p. 88). Eat wholegrains, which should make up around 35 percent of your daily diet, rather than refined alternatives such as white bread, rice, and some pasta.

Nuts and seeds are an important source of antioxidants – the vitamins and minerals that help prevent molecules known as free radicals from damaging cell function. Sprouted seeds such as alfalfa, mung, and soybeans, and also oats, buckwheat, and wheatgrass, are high in antioxidant vitamins C, A, and E, and also B vitamins, proteins, and possibly important enzymes. Nuts are high in calcium, magnesium, and zinc, and Brazil nuts are high in selenium, an important antioxidant mineral.

High-energy grains, nuts, and seeds include: brown rice, wholewheat and rye bread, durum wheat pasta, oatmeal, buckwheat, maize, Brazil nuts, sesame and sunflower seeds, and sprouted seeds.

Proteins High-protein foods include poultry, white fish, shellfish, eggs, and low-fat dairy products. Red meat and full-cream dairy products are also high in protein, but have a high saturated fat content. Pulses such as lentils, beans, peas, and seeds are not only a great source of protein but are also slow-releasing carbohydrates, which means they do not cause a rapid rise in blood sugar. For high energy, cut down on red meat and high-fat dairy produce, which are much less easily digested. Protein should make up around 15 percent of your daily diet, but vegetable proteins don't give high energy, so if you are vegan, get your protein from cereals, nuts, and seeds.

High-protein foods include: peas, beans, lentils, chickpeas, chicken, white fish such as haddock and seabass, soya milk, low-fat yogurt, and sprouted seeds.

Essential fatty acids (EFAs) A special mention in the high-energy food group goes to EFAs. These are obtained only from the food we eat; our body cannot manufacture them. The two most important EFAs are linoleic acid (an omega 6 fatty acid) and alpha-linolenic acid (an omega 3 fatty acid). They are involved in the manufacture of sex hormones and prostaglandins, chemicals that are vital to the immune system response, and are especially important during pregnancy for fetal brain development and to protect against premature birth. EFAs are essential for our growth and development, and they may help to reduce the symptoms of depression and lower the risk of heart attack. A lack of EFAs is thought to compromise the immune system, and the health of the heart, brain, skin, hair, and nails.

Foods high in omega 6 EFAs include: sunflower, sesame, and pumpkin seeds, almonds, walnuts, soybeans, linseed (flax), sunflower and rapeseed oil. Arachidonic acid, another omega 6 EFA, is present in oily fish (sardines, mackerel), meat, and dairy products.

Foods high in omega 3 EFAs include: oily fish, evening primrose and blackcurrant seed oils, linseed and rapeseed oil, walnuts, pumpkin seeds, and soybeans.

Fats An essential element in our diet, fat not only ensures sufficient EFAs, but is an important source of energy and vitamins, and it keeps us warm. Many of us eat a diet deficient in fat, afraid that we might put on weight.

Eat fats from: vegetable oils (olive, sunflower, linseed), oily fish, nuts, and seeds, rather than from saturated (animal) fats.

Recommended Daily Allowances (RDAs)

RDAs are a guide based on the minimal needs of a healthy adult (larger quantities of some vitamins may be beneficial). Here are the RDAs of some energy vitamins:

Vitamin C. 60 mg. Found in many fruit and vegetables.

Iron. 18 mg. Found in eggs, meat, dairy produce, leafy green vegetables.

Calcium. 1 g. Found in dairy products, eggs, peas, dried beans.

Vitamin B1. 1.5 mg. Found in meat, wholegrains, peas.

Regular meals mean high energy

It may sound simple, but it is vital to eat regularly to maintain good energy levels. As we have discussed (see p. 28), many of us skip meals because of poor time management, a misplaced desire to reduce calorie intake, or because we are buying into the general disrespect for food that sadly has become part of our culture. But by skipping meals we are ignoring what our body is telling us it needs, and thus at risk of inadequate nutrition and erratic blood sugar levels. This leads to fatigue, mood swings, binge eating and drinking, a compromised immune system and, over time, can result in weight gain and even diabetes.

The sugar seesaw It works like this. When you starve yourself your blood sugar level drops and you become tired and irritable. This triggers a craving for something sweet to raise your blood sugar quickly, so you probably reach for a chocolate bar or cookie. The quick carbohydrate hit satisfies you temporarily by driving up your blood sugar level. But to deal with the rapid rise of sugar and prevent too much accumulating in the bloodstream, your body has to produce a lot of insulin, which metabolizes the sugar and drives your blood sugar back down to where it was before you ate the chocolate. So what do you do? Eat another cookie, and the whole cycle begins again. Many people spend their days on this seesaw of poor nutrition.

Eating regular, moderately sized meals, starting with breakfast of course, will avoid this vicious cycle. If you do have to delay a meal, snack on slow-releasing carbohydrates (see p. 86) such as wholegrain products, nuts, fruit, and dried fruit that raise blood sugar more slowly and maintain a healthy balance.

The glycemic index scale

The glycemic index scale is a way of measuring the effect that the carbohydrate content in certain foods has on blood sugar levels; it is a measure of how quickly and to what extent sugar is released into the bloodstream compared with pure glucose, which is rated at 100. The lower the score the better.

The scale is used in a new diet idea that aims to combat the sugar seesaw described above. There is also a belief, which Barry Sears describes in his diet book *The Zone*, that slow-releasing carbohydrates, which score low on the glycemic index, should be balanced with an increased protein intake; this is because glucagon, a hormone secreted by the pancreas that balances the effect of insulin, is triggered by protein in the diet.

Low glycemic index foods include: lentils, chickpeas, peanuts, pears, dried apricots, plums, grapefruit, porridge oats, yogurt, and wholemeal spaghetti.

The anti-candida diet

There is a growing but controversial belief by some nutritionists that low energy may be due to yeast *(Candida albicans)* overgrowth in the intestine. The anti-candida diet is very difficult to follow unless you prepare your own food, and undertaken without expert supervision it can lead to nutritional deficiencies. The diet involves eliminating sugars and yeast-containing foods and is therefore very restrictive indeed; it means no white flour or potatoes, for example. To find out more about this diet and potential supplements, read John Briffa's book *Ultimate Health*.

FOOD TIPS FOR HIGH ENERGY

- Eat a wide variety of foods to gain the maximum nutrients.
- Read labels and sell-by dates; avoid foods containing high numbers of additives and/or preservatives.
- Steam or stir-fry vegetables to preserve the nutrients.
- Eat regular, moderately sized meals and never skip a meal, particularly breakfast; snack often.
- Eat fresh, unprocessed food, and lots of fruit and vegetables.
- Wash fruit and vegetables thoroughly to remove pesticides.
- For sustained energy, eat slow-releasing carbohydrates.
- Avoid stimulants such as alcohol and caffeine, high sugar, high. saturated fat, and high-salt food. Replace salt with herbal alternatives.
- Make time to enjoy eating; never eat when you're upset or stressed.
- Drink 1.5–2 quarts (1.5–2 liters) of pure mineral or filtered water every day.

Vitamins and supplements

To supplement or not to supplement, that is the question! Nutritionists are divided about whether vitamin and mineral supplements are necessary or simply a waste of money. Most people in the Western world do suffer serious vitamin deficiencies, and consume levels of nutrients that do not encourage high energy. Carefully targeted supplementation seems to be the answer.

We cannot make the vitamins that are present in food, especially fruit and vegetables. Vitamins are essential for the growth and maintenance of healthy body tissues. They do not provide energy themselves, but act as enzymes that regulate the production of energy and nutrients that the body needs for its normal metabolism.

Vitamin depletion The average modern diet rarely supplies enough vitamins. Food quality has been compromised; intensive farming, for example, robs the soil of nutrients, and we eat too many processed foods. And toxins such as caffeine, alcohol, and tobacco increase our needs for vitamins and minerals.

Should we supplement? Of course! Most of us are unlikely to eat a perfect, balanced diet, so it makes sense to take a multivitamin and mineral supplement, an essential fatty acid (EFA) supplement, and also to consider taking some of the herbal energy-boosters detailed below.

Vitamin and mineral supplements are only part of a healthy diet, not a substitute for good food. So the best policy is eat healthily and supplement moderately.

Which supplements do we need? Our needs differ depending on diet, age, and lifestyle. To find out exactly which supplements your body needs, testing by a qualified nutritionist may guide you, or you might consult a qualified healthcare practitioner. Some products contain very little of the active ingredient or use poor quality capsules. You'll get what you pay for!

Energy-boosting supplements

Over and above general dietary supplementation, additional supplementation to improve energy levels should be considered only after you have addressed the underlying causes of your low energy and eliminated lifestyle or medical factors. However, following a period of difficulty or stress, or recovering from illness, you may need an energy boost. Try some of the following energy pick-me-ups:

Coenzyme Q10 (CoQ10) Present in all body cells, CoQ10 is necessary for cellular energy production. It is a powerful antioxidant, said to boost immunity, sperm health, physical performance, and is important to heart health and in the prevention of cancer.
Dietary sources include: wholegrains, nuts, green vegetables, meat, and fish.

L-carnitine An amino acid made in the liver, L-carnitine is important for fat metabolism and energy production. It may also reduce fatigue and is known to increase oxygen uptake in muscles, resulting in more stamina. L-carnitine is helpful in heart disease and in chronic fatigue syndrome.
Dietary sources include: red meat, dairy products, and avocado pears.
Side effects: high doses may have a laxative effect.

HOW TO TAKE SUPPLEMENTS

To avoid nausea, it is usually the rule to take supplements immediately after food unless otherwise stated, and to take them with water or fruit juice. Coffee and tea should not be drunk with supplements, as they can hinder absorption of some vitamins and minerals, such as iron, zinc, calcium, and some B vitamins. Smoking also reduces the absorption of vitamin C.

If you are taking a number of supplements, spread them out over the day, but avoid taking B complex vitamins at night as they may interfere with sleep. Always follow the manufacturer's instructions regarding dose, unless you are under professional supervision.

Supplements will not be as beneficial if they are taken erratically, so try and get into a routine where you take them at the same time every day.

Siberian ginseng (*Eleutherococcus senticosus*) Known as an adaptogen because it helps the body adapt under stress. This can relieve anxiety or increase stamina, and ease menopausal symptoms. No dietary source.

Side effects: negligible, but do not take it if you have high blood pressure, tachycardia (rapid heartbeat), heart failure, or heavy periods.

Guarana (*Paullinia cupana*) A quick lift for mental and physical energy levels, guarana contains naturally slow-released caffeine. Taken regularly over some weeks, it is said to reduce stress, aid the immune system, and ease premenstrual syndrome and period pains. No dietary source.

Side effects: some people experience caffeine-related symptoms.

Royal jelly Secreted by worker bees and full of vitamins and minerals, this is a real energy tonic. It reduces stress, boosts vitality, relieves tiredness and sleeplessness, and improves the condition of skin, hair, and nails. No dietary source.

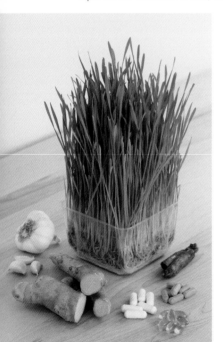

Side effects: can trigger an asthma attack in those allergic to bee pollen.

Energy-boosting vitamins and minerals

The following vitamin and mineral supplements are good general health and energy-boosters:

Vitamin C If you take no other supplement, take this one. A powerful antioxidant, it boosts the immune system and taking at least 1 g a day protects against disease. It is vital for tissue repair and iron absorption. Deficiency causes slow wound healing, bleeding gums, and weakness.

"Eat healthily and supplement moderately" should be the maxim for high energy.

Dietary sources include: citrus fruits, green leafy vegetables, and blackcurrants.
Side effects: high doses can have a laxative effect.

Vitamin B complex includes vitamins B1, B2, B3, B5, B6, and B12. These work best taken together. Important in metabolism, energy production, and enzyme function, they also improve brain function and therefore influence mood.
Dietary sources include: wholegrains, nuts, eggs, meat, and green leafy vegetables.
Side effects: taken in high doses, B3 may cause flushing and B6 (over 150 mg daily) can cause nerve and liver damage.

Calcium An important mineral for bones and teeth, and vital for blood clotting, the conduction of nerve impulses, energy production, and immune system function. Deficiency can lead to osteoporosis, particularly in women. No side effects.
Dietary sources include: most plant foods, nuts, seeds, dairy products, and pulses.

Magnesium This is vital in energy production, healthy nerve cell function, the metabolism of EFAs, and the production of mood chemicals such as dopamine. Deficiency can cause tiredness, loss of appetite, muscle weakness, and palpitations.
Dietary sources include: wholegrains, dark-green leafy vegetables, and seafood.
Side effects: large doses can cause diarrhea.

Zinc This trace mineral is vital for immunity, insulin activity, growth, wound healing, and sex hormone function. Deficiency can cause weak hair and nails, loss of taste, smell, and appetite, and skin conditions.
Dietary sources include: shellfish, red meat, wholegrains, pulses, eggs, and cheese.
Side effects: do not take high doses (over 30 mg daily) for long periods without medical advice.

Probiotic supplements These are important when taking antibiotics (see p. 69). They replace "friendly" bacteria, including bifidobacteria and lactobacilli, which are eradicated along with harmful bacteria by antibiotics. Take 1–2 billion CFUs of acidophilus per dose for several weeks. No side effects.
Dietary sources include: Live "bio" yogurts and fermented milk drinks.

Liquid energy (juicing)

Liquid energy is a quick and easy way to consume vitamins and minerals. Herbal teas, freshly squeezed juice, "smoothies," and blended energy drinks are obvious, readily available choices if you need a healthy pick-me-up during your busy day.

Juicing for instant vitality Raw juices are a great instant energy hit. Squeezing or pressing fruit and vegetables to drink has become a popular way to ingest nutrients and it provides the benefits of raw food without having to chew it. But don't be tempted to take all your fresh produce in this way; your body also needs the flesh of the fruit and vegetables for bulk and fiber.

Top tips for top-quality juice

■ Buy a juicer that's easy to clean and assemble and you'll use it more often.

■ Juice with organic fruit and vegetables; concentrated pressed juice means concentrated pesticides and chemicals, too.

■ Wash all fruit and vegetables thoroughly before juicing.

■ Buy the freshest fruit and vegetables you can find and use them as soon as possible; avoid underripe or overripe produce.

■ To gain maximum nutrient benefit, try as wide a variety as possible of fruit and vegetable combinations.

■ Drink the juice as soon it's squeezed or it will lose a lot of valuable enzymes.

All-day energy in a glass

Here is a selection of easy-to-make energy drinks that help provide day-long vitality:

Breakfast cocktail In her *Encyclopaedia of Vitamins and Minerals*, Dr. Sarah Brewer recommends this high-energy pick-me-up made from the Brazilian plant, guarana: mix a teaspoon (5 ml) each of guarana powder, brewer's yeast, and wheatgerm in a glass with 15 ml of pure, organic honey, then top it up with mineral water. Mix thoroughly and drink every morning before breakfast.

Mid-morning boost Squeeze a lemon and pour the juice into a glass. Add a tablespoon of honey and top it up with sparkling mineral water to taste.

Evening cocktail Juice two large tomatoes and squeeze the juice of half a lemon, add a teaspoon of tamari (a dark sauce made from soybeans), a pinch of thyme, herb salt, and Tabasco to taste. Stir and drink chilled.

Evening calmer Place one ¾ in (2 cm) long stick of cinnamon, or one teaspoon of ground cinnamon, and 8 fl oz (200 ml) of rice milk into a saucepan. Bring to the boil and simmer gently for a couple of minutes. Pour into a mug and add honey to taste. Drink immediately.

Caffeine substitutes

Be it tea or coffee, the caffeine habit is a difficult one to break, not least because of the pleasure we derive when we drink a cup with friends. But instead of using coffee beans, try dandelion or chicory "coffee," green tea, herbal infusions, or try brewing up a root tea with ginger.

Dandelion root (*Taraxacum officinalis*) This is a good, general detoxifier, it has a gentle diuretic and laxative effect, and helps with the absorption of iron. It also acts as a mild tonic.

Chicory root (*Cichorium intybus*) This tastes more bitter than coffee, but has been used for centuries as a digestive. Like coffee, the root is dried, roasted, and then ground.

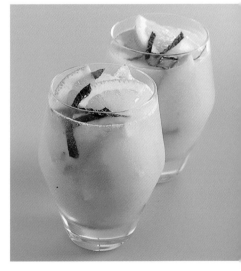

Green tea This has been drunk by the Chinese for thousands of years, not just because it is refreshing, cleansing, and mildly stimulating, but also for its antioxidant qualities. Brew it like ordinary tea and drink without milk.

Ginger root (*Zingiber officinale*) Ginger has many health benefits. It has analgesic

For a boost, try fresh-squeezed fruit and vegetable juice.

(painkilling) and antihistamine properties, it stimulates the circulation, and helps prevent nausea. Ginger root infusion is a good digestive to drink after a meal: Take half an inch of root ginger, peel it, slice it thinly, and put it in a small saucepan with two large cups of water. Bring to the boil, cover, and simmer gently for five minutes, strain, and serve.

RECIPES FOR HIGH-ENERGY JUICING

Any combination of fruit and vegetables is acceptable, depending on your tastes, but here are a few combinations to set you off:

RECIPE ONE

1 apple, peeled and cored

1 pear, peeled and cored

2 carrots

1 small cube of ginger root, peeled

1 orange, squeezed

Juice the apple, pear, carrots, and ginger, and then add the squeezed orange juice.

RECIPE TWO

½ a mango, peeled and stoned

¼ a pineapple, peeled

½ a banana, peeled

3 lychees, peeled and stoned

1 orange, squeezed

Juice the fruits and add the squeezed orange juice.

Or, for variety, you can make a high-energy smoothie, adding soy or almond milk to your pressed fruits.

RECIPE THREE

4 fresh apricots, stoned

1 banana, peeled

1½ fl oz (50 ml) almond milk

1 pinch of cinnamon

Blend the fruits and milk, and stir in the cinnamon.

RECIPE FOUR

1 banana, peeled

1 chunk of fresh coconut

3½ fl oz (100 ml) soy milk

1 teaspoon of honey

Blend all the ingredients together and serve chilled.

Herbal infusions

Because stress is one of the major factors in depleting energy, it makes good sense to substitute coffee and tea containing stress-inducing caffeine with herbal infusions. The stressful effects of caffeine include palpitations, anxiety, and disturbed sleep patterns.

Herbal infusions, or "teas," such as the ones listed below are an excellent substitute and have positive benefits for your health and energy, too.

For all the herbal infusions, steep the fresh or dried herb in boiling water for about 10 minutes, strain, and serve without milk.

Chamomile (*Matricaria chamomilla*) This reduces anxiety and has a mild, sedative effect as well as antiinflammatory and antispasmodic properties. It also helps to relieve skin irritation. Drink this infusion before you go to bed to help you sleep well.

Passionflower (*Passiflora incarnata*) Passionflower relieves anxiety and mild nerve pain such as neuralgia. It also helps you to sleep.

Fennel (*Foeniculum vulgare*) Fennel is what is known as a carminative; this means that it relieves gas and generally soothes the digestion. It can be made into a warm infusion by using either the herb or the crushed seeds.

(Recipes adapted from Energize Your Life *by Nic Rowley, Kirsten Hartvig, Emma Mitchell and Alistair Livingstone.)*

Dips and Spreads with Essential Fatty Acids

In Liz Earle's book *New Vital Oils* she suggests some easy ways to include EFAs – the oils vital for energy and boosting your immune system – in your diet. Try this dip to eat with fresh, raw vegetable sticks. Mix low-fat soft cheese or yogurt with flavoring such as lemon juice, Tabasco sauce, chopped herbs, and garlic, then stir in 1 tablespoon (15 ml) of hazlenut or walnut oil.

Or make a spread for bread or rice cakes by adding a teaspoon each of oil, such as olive, pumpkin, or sunflower, to low-fat soft cheese or cottage cheese, and seasoning with celery salt and cayenne pepper to taste.

relaxation

Living a rushed and stressful life can become a habit. Because stress is so destructive to our energy levels, we need to learn about the different mechanisms that can help to reduce it if we want to achieve optimum vitality. This involves mind-calming techniques, exercise to flush the stress hormones from the body, and suggestions to help ensure a refreshing night's sleep.

Meditation

Many studies have been carried out on the effects of meditation and they all show that regular meditation can reduce anxiety, stress, and depression, and encourages self-awareness, a clear mind, and it even helps lower blood pressure. Don't be put off by its sometimes hippy image; being able to disappear into a calm place in your head is a fantastic antidote for our highly stressful lives.

Brain waves During meditation, brain activity shifts from the normal alert, waking state, characterized by beta waves, to the slower more meditative levels, characterized by alpha, theta, and the lowest level of brain activity, delta waves.

Delta vibrations are experienced in very deep sleep or in a meditative state where we are unaware of the world around us. As a result of slowing the mind but remaining conscious, we can access the brain's vast potential and become detached from petty thoughts and worries. This detachment allows us a perspective on self and life that, over time, can help us become calm and mentally strong.

A simple meditation technique Vipassana, a form of meditation, was developed by the Tibetan Buddhists and the technique it employs is wonderfully simple. There is no success or failure in any meditation, just practice, so don't be tempted to judge your performance. The first few times you meditate may well seem useless and chaotic but just keep trying. Here's what to do:

- Set aside 10–20 minutes, ideally always at the same time, every day.
- Find a warm, quiet place with no phones, people, or other distractions.
- Sit comfortably on a chair, or cross-legged on the floor.
- Sit straight by imagining a string from the center of your head is pulling you up.
- Relax your muscles both internally and externally.
- Breathing gently in and out through your nose, close your eyes and concentrate on your breath in, and your breath out. Feel the air entering and leaving your body.

Start with 10 minutes and build up to 20 as it comes more naturally. At first your thoughts will probably crowd in and distract you; simply acknowledge each thought briefly, as if it were a performer on stage, then say good-bye as you watch it drift off stage and disappear. Return to your breathing. Do this with every intrusive thought and, after a while, you will enjoy a sense of calm.

After 10 minutes, open your eyes and take a couple of deep breaths; you will feel refreshed. With practice, you will access more and more of your inner self, and in moments of stress or panic you will know a place where you can be still.

Visualization

Visualization is a form of meditation that can be used for problem solving and for body healing. The belief is that regular visualization prompts the body to react to the positive, visualized scenario rather than the less pleasant reality, and that this reduces anxiety and promotes healing. Visualization is now accepted by many cancer and AIDS specialists as powerful medicine.

De-stress with visualization If you are feeling stressed, try this:

- Sit comfortably, as you would to meditate (see above).
- Imagine you are in beautiful, natural surroundings. It can be somewhere real or imagined, but it is safe and special to you. Breath the air, feel the breeze on your cheek, the sunlight on your face, see the colors, smell the earth. Breathe gently and relax into the image as if you were there.
- Stay in this magic place for 15 minutes, then open your eyes and take a couple of deep breaths. You will feel calm and at peace. Return to this image whenever you are upset or wound up; you can also use the technique to help you sleep.

Breathing

If we do not breathe, we die, and yet we are rarely conscious of breathing; it is an automatic function. However, by training ourselves to breathe much more efficiently we can feel calmer and enhance our energy levels as well as our ability to heal.

Breathing for energy For our body systems to function well, we need a good supply of oxygen that we obtain from the air we breathe. Put simply, breathing takes in oxygen and eliminates carbon dioxide. So, the more efficiently we breathe, the better our carbon dioxide/oxygen balance, the more alert, less tired and stressed, and the less vulnerable to disease we will be.

Deep diaphragmatic breathing slows the brain waves from beta to alpha, it slows the heart rate, and we feel calmer. "Take a deep breath" is not a common imperative for nothing; breathing deeply can be the first line of defense against panic attacks, anxiety, and any stressful situation.

Break bad habits Over a lifetime we breathe in and out around half a billion times. But many of us breathe too fast, too erratically, and too high in our chest, instead of deeply from the diaphragm to fill our lungs full.

Shallow, inadequate breathing upsets the carbon dioxide/oxygen balance in our body and zaps our energy.

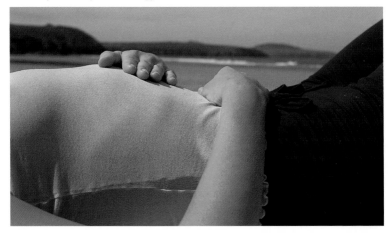

Some of us have acquired a breathing technique which encourages what stress counselor Dr. David Lewis calls "upside-down breathing," in which we use mainly the secondary breathing muscles in the upper chest instead of the diaphragm. This shallow breathing does not fully expand the lungs to allow maximum oxygen intake.

There are a number of reasons for failing to breathe deeply:

- As a child copies talking, so it copies breathing.
- Poor posture; if we are hunched or slumped over, the chest cannot fully expand.
- Tight clothes or holding in your stomach makes for shallow breathing.
- Stress and tension cause fast and shallow breathing.

Breathe through your nose The cilia (tiny hairs) lining the nose filter pollutants such as smoke, bacteria, dust, and pollen, by wafting them to the back of the throat from where they are coughed out, or swallowed and eliminated via the intestine. The mucous membrane in the nose moistens and warms inhaled air before it reaches the delicate lung tissue.

Take a deep breath Deep, diaphragmatic breathing for two – five minutes each day retrains your body to breathe correctly and leaves you feeling relaxed.

- Lie on the floor, knees flexed, arms by your sides.
- Inhale slowly and deeply through your nose, arching the small of your back a few inches off the floor and saying "in" silently to yourself. Feel the breath enter your nose and travel slowly via your throat to expand your chest and lungs.
- Breathe out gently through your nose, pressing the small of your back into the floor. Say "out" silently to yourself as the breath is slowly exhaled from your body.

Energizing cleansing breath Kapalabhati is a cleansing breath that also gives the body an energy boost. Do this quickly 20 times and repeat three cycles:

- Sit on the floor with your legs crossed, hands on your knees.
- Sharply contract your stomach muscles to forcefully exhale through your nose.
- Allow the breath to flow effortlessly back through the nose into the lungs.

As well as learning how to breathe, make a habit of standing and sitting tall with your chest open and shoulders relaxed. Regular exercise also encourages good, full lung expansion as you take big, deep breaths.

Sleep

People who sleep easily and deeply have more energy. But many of us toss and turn night after night, nodding off for what feels like only five minutes before the alarm clock rings. Sleeplessness is a profound energy drainer.

Insomnia We all have disrupted nights occasionally, but research shows that our bodies usually adapt and eventually right the balance with good, deep sleep.

But when lack of sleep becomes the norm, instead of looking forward to going to bed we dread the whole process, knowing even before our head hits the pillow that long hours of tense wakefulness lie ahead. And the harder you try to get to sleep, the less likely you are to do so.

Persistent insomnia raises stress levels, reduces our energy, and predisposes to depressed immunity and even heart attacks.

More worry, less sleep How we think about our sleep is vital. The more rigid you are about how much sleep you need, the more stressed you will be about not getting it. So relax. Research shows that even diehard insomniacs sleep more than they think they do. Instead of tossing and turning, get up and read or listen to soothing music for half an hour.

Contain your worries. If you can't sort them out, put them on hold with this mantra: "Nothing can be resolved during the hours of darkness." Write your worries down before you go to bed and leave them on the kitchen table to be dealt with in the morning. If you find yourself churning over them, repeat the mantra three times.

Monitor bad habits Drink less coffee, alcohol, and tea, and smoke fewer cigarettes late at night. Eat lightly in the evening, and avoid sugary foods late at night that might give you a sugar high just when you need calming down. Drink warm milk, but don't add chocolate! Don't watch overstimulating TV late at night.

Exercise during the day to burn off stress hormones and release endorphins, the body's natural opiates. An evening walk, even a short one, can also help you sleep.

Regulate your sleeping habits – sleep clinics make much of this. Go to bed and get up at the same time each day, and establish a routine before bed, as you would for a baby, so that your mind and body are prepared for the concept of sleep.

Techniques to help you sleep We hold tension in our bodies unconsciously, so try this relaxation technique when you are lying in bed: starting with your toes and working up your body, tense each muscle group for the count of three, and then release; include even finger and face muscles. Your body should now feel very relaxed. You could try three minutes of deep, diaphragmatic breathing (see p. 101), or ask your partner to massage your neck and shoulders with a lavender-based aromatherapy oil for five minutes before bed.

Prepare for a good night's sleep

The quality of what you sleep on, under, and in is vital for a good night's sleep:

■ The mattress should be firm but comfortable. And, according to the Chinese philosophy, feng shui, the bed should face north.

■ Pillows should not be too fat or hard; covers should keep you warm not sweaty.

■ Nightclothes should be neither voluminous nor restrictive.

■ The bedroom should be well aired, dark, and as quiet as possible.

■ Reduce to a minimum electronic equipment in the bedroom.

■ Keep water at your bedside.

Complementary remedies If none of the measures discussed so far have helped, then you might try one of the following sleep remedies:

Lavender essential oil Sprinkle a few drops of lavender essential oil on your pillow, or before bed take a warm bath – not hot, because that may stimulate you – containing lavender oil.

Nux vomica and belladonna This remedy is recommended by Dr. Mosaraf Ali for stress-related insomnia. Put two tablets of nux vomica 200C on the tongue at bedtime, then five minutes later add two tablets of belladonna 30C on the tongue. This high-potency (200C) of nux vomica should be taken only under the supervision of a qualified homeopath.

Valerian Drink a cup of valerian tea before bed, or take 10–15 valeriana drops in a quarter of a cup of water.

Acupuncture This therapy can reduce anxiety and aid sleep.

If you remain troubled by persistent insomnia, consult your doctor, but beware of drugs that induce dependency. In extremis, you may be referred to a sleep clinic.

Exercise

Exercise is not just about burning calories. Our bodies are designed to move and if we don't keep active we stiffen up, our bodies ache and get out of shape, both outside and in. There are many different forms of exercise to choose from, and it is important to find one that you enjoy and that fits in with your way of life.

Be realistic Exercise is one of the best ways to boost energy and self-esteem. To find which form, or forms, of exercise will suit you best, try a few different options rather than commit to something in haste. Make sure that whatever you choose is realistic. Don't buy a mountain bike if you'll never ride it.

The benefits of exercise

There are three types of exercise:

Aerobic exercise causes the heart rate to rise and the body to use oxygen to convert fat into energy, such as when you jog, swim, or dance.

Anaerobic exercise is when the body uses glycogen already stored in the muscles during short, intense bursts of activity, such as jumping, sprinting, or lifting.

Stretching exercise such as yoga, Pilates, or tai chi does not increase heart rate.

Cross-training This combines different forms of exercise and is ideal for overall fitness because you work your body differently with each one. For example, a good mix would be one half-hour swim, two walks, and a yoga class – combining aerobic and stretching exercise – and would take no more than four hours a week.

Interval training Used by athletes to increase stamina and enhance fitness, interval training is based on varying the intensity of cardiovascular activity for short intervals during a workout. It uses the time you are exercising to best advantage, burns more calories, and spices up what could become a dull grind.

Rate your exercise on a scale from 1 (least active) to 10 (most active): slow walking rates 2–3, brisk walking rates 4–6, a burst of anaerobic exercise, such as a quick sprint, rates 7–10. During a workout – be it swimming, jogging, cycling – include spurts of anaerobic activity: walk briskly (4–6), then sprint for one or two minutes (7–10), then walk slowly (2–3). Repeat the sequence as often as you want.

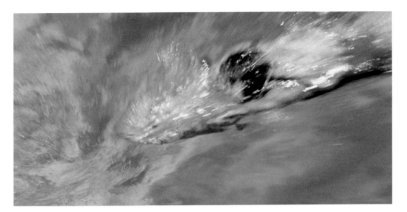

Use interval training to spice up your exercise routine and increase your cardiovascular fitness.

Motivation Competitive team sports such as tennis, softball, or soccer have the advantage of involving other people to spur you on and encourage you. And, if you don't like the idea of exercise as "training," you can focus on the game. Or join a dance class. Music is a great motivator and dancing involves stretching and fluid movement as well as aerobic exercise.

Warm up, cool down Don't leap into any strenuous activity without first warming up for five minutes; this guards against muscle injury. Warm up with a stretching sequence, or a gentle version of the exercise, to loosen up your muscles and ligaments. For the last five minutes of your workout, reduce the level of activity, or finish with a stretching sequence involving hamstrings, calves, and quadriceps.

Know your limit Don't overdo a new exercise regime, or you risk straining your body. Drink plenty of water to prevent dehydration, and wear suitable shoes and clothing for the exercise.

Never push yourself beyond your limit. To improve aerobic fitness you should be out of breath but still able to hold a conversation without difficulty, not gasping and unable to speak. If your breathing rate regularly takes more than five minutes to return to normal, consult your doctor.

Exercise for mind-body balance

Mind, body, spirit philosophies that originate in the East, such as yoga and tai chi, are designed to balance the whole body, internally and externally. So, as well as improving physical strength and flexibility, these philosophies are great stress busters.

Eastern exercise forms are progressive so that you go on learning and improving your movement, meditation, and breathing skills over a lifetime.

Yoga

An ancient philosophy and system of movement with its roots in India, yoga was devised to combine all aspects of body, mind, and spirit to encourage spiritual enlightenment. It has gained popularity in the West as a gentle way to tone, strengthen, and mobilize the body for people of all ages, but practiced regularly yoga also calms the mind and greatly enhances spiritual well-being. It is a good antidote to the chaotic, aspiritual life so many of us lead.

Energy balance According to Eastern philosophy, an energy network, known as subtle energy, or prana, runs through the body via paths (nadis), and through seven energy centers (the chakras). The chakras, starting at the base of the torso, are called "base," "sacral," "solar plexus," "heart," "throat," "third eye," and "crown." When you are ill or have low energy, it is because your subtle energy is blocked and out of balance. Regular yoga practice can help to right the balance.

Asanas are the poses that, in conjunction with breathwork, bring about yogic balance. Each pose stretches and strengthens the muscles improving tone and flexibility, but poses are also said to benefit body organs and calm the mind.

Movement and meditation Of yoga's many different branches the most commonly practiced in the West is hatha yoga. This centers on postural movements (asanas), breathwork (pranayama), and meditation (dyana). Versions of hatha yoga include: astanga, popularized as "power yoga," Iyengar, which involves very precise physical poses and breathwork, and sivananda, which involves chanting, meditation, spiritual teaching, and diet.

Whichever form of yoga you choose, it is best to learn from a qualified teacher at a yoga center that offers graded classes depending on previous experience.

Martial arts

All the martial arts aim to improve mental, physical, and spiritual strength, but they fall into two categories: "soft" martial arts, such as tai chi, focus on the internal body system; "hard" martial arts, such as kung fu, focus on the external body.

Tai chi Qigong, or "working with energy," is the overall term for the numerous ancient Chinese movement systems, of which tai chi is but one. A martial art based on Taoist philosophy, tai chi is also a mind, body, spirit exercise form that, like yoga, aims to make the body stronger and more flexible while freeing its energy pathways, so that qi, the Chinese equivalent of prana, can flow unimpeded.

Tai chi involves a series of poses linked with graceful, fluid movements and has been termed a "moving meditation." It is concerned with relaxation, balance, and grounding the body, the feet in contact with the earth, so that qi can travel through the body from the torso to the head and limbs.

Research has shown tai chi to be an excellent discipline for reducing stress and anxiety. You will need to learn this ancient art from a qualified teacher as it involves breathwork and meditation as well as many different postures.

Martial arts provide a workout for mind, body, and spirit, and are more mentally challenging than purely sports-based exercise.

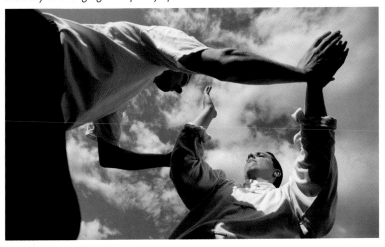

Stress and the psychospiritual

If life is an unfulfilling grind, just working to pay the bills, you are unconsciously living with stress that is depleting your energy. Even continual boredom is stressful. It is important, therefore, to find purpose in life, and to set personal goals that are unconnected to the acquisition of material wealth, and that instead address your emotional and spiritual development.

The stress of isolation Despite being surrounded by people, we can feel lonely and isolated. The elderly, the sick, or anyone who stands out as "different" can feel isolated, which can create stress and unhappiness. We can feel isolated within a family, among friends, or at work, when we feel we are not understood. The result is the same – stress and unhappiness.

Best friends? For whatever reason – economic perhaps, or a misplaced sense of social aspiration, or simply the habit of a friendship long past its sell-by date – we may align ourselves with people, socially and at work, who are not sympathetic to who we really are. But every moment you spend with people who do not make you feel good is a moment you should try and cut from your life.

Energy vampires Through no fault of their own, some of your friends may be "energy vampires." They drain your energy but give nothing in return: their plans are chaotic, they're usually late, they always talk about themselves never about you, they need you to be their rock.

We all have to make compromises sometimes, but we should reduce the times that we do. Take a moment to review the people with whom you hang out. Do you come away from these meetings feeling energized, listened to, and full of self-esteem? Or do you come away feeling insecure, exhausted, and put down?

Believe in yourself To "be yourself" might seem obvious, but many people live under the strain of being the person that others expect them to be. This can make them resentful, especially if they don't feel validated. This way of being might even extend to the work that they do. It may stem from a childhood where their personality was lost becuse of parental expectations.

Assuming you have only one life, don't wait too long to live it. If there is an aspect of your life that makes you unhappy, even if it's having only a little time to yourself each week, make changes that will suit you better. No one else will!

A healthy respect for spirituality

Everyone has a spirit, that indefinable element that connects us to a universal consciousness and is much deeper than mind and body. However, our spirit is often drowned out by today's secular, material world. Whatever your belief, having a spiritual dimension to your life has been shown to be extremely beneficial. It guides you, makes you feel protected, gives your life purpose, connects you with others, reduces stress, and even helps your body to recover more quickly from illness.

Finding inner peace and calm So how, if you do not belong to a religion or faith, do you access your spirit? The answer is that it is within us all, and to find it we have to still the mind, putting our conscious brain on hold, and looking inward until we feel it.

This can be done in a number of different ways, so we can all find a path to spirituality that appeals to our sensibility. You might turn to a defined spiritual practice, such as religion, prayer, or meditation. You might do as many ancient cultures have done, and find the universal spirit in art, dance, drumming, music, or chanting. You might use the angel world to connect and guide you. You might find it in exercise techniques such as yoga, tai chi, or breathing.

Try connecting with the spirit force within you and you will find a place of peace where you can grow spiritually, calm your mind, and find purpose to your life. High energy will be harder to find if your mind and spirit are in turmoil.

Live life for the moment Mindfulness is a Buddhist concept about living in the moment. Our reality is the here and now, yet many of us live perpetually in either the past or the future, never really enjoying all that we have, the present moment.

Mindfulness is not an easy thing to achieve but it is well worth practicing. Even if you are doing a mundane task, such as washing, focus all your energies into what you are doing, and do it as perfectly as you can. You will find the practice helps to stop anxious thoughts and will bring great satisfaction and peace of mind.

complementary

therapies

Complementary medicine has become increasingly popular as people in the West are beginning to understand what Eastern healing philosophies have always accepted: disease is not simply a set of symptoms that occur at random, but an intricate warning system alerting us to deeper imbalances in our homeostasis. There is a growing realization that prevention is better than cure, and that by monitoring and looking after our health we can avoid disease.

Conventional medicine has a vital part to play in the battle against disease, but taking an integrated approach, which uses complementary therapies in conjunction with conventional medicine, is surely the best way to achieve and maintain good health.

This section looks at what complementary therapies can offer, and which should best address your needs.

body
alignment

Therapies that rebalance the body's structure are also restorative to energy levels. This section looks at different complementary therapies we can employ to realign our bodies when they have been damaged or put out of kilter. They include manipulative therapies, such as osteopathy and massage, exercise disciplines such as Pilates and the Alexander Technique, and healing arts such as acupuncture and reflexology.

Manipulative therapies

As well as rebalancing body alignment, the manipulative therapies discussed here are holistic in nature and are restorative both to general health and to energy levels.

Osteopathy

One of the most popular complementary therapies, osteopathy is not only effective in treating structural problems, it can also help with headaches, digestive and respiratory problems, sinusitis, and menstrual dysfunction.

How does it work? The technique of osteopathy was devised by an American doctor, Andrew Taylor Still, in 1874. He believed that illness was partially a result of structural misalignment and that if the skeleton was out of kilter it would cause inflammation in the nearby muscles and tissue. This in turn would affect the smooth flow of blood around the body, thereby disrupting the immune system and thus resulting in disease.

Misalignment of the body might happen as a result of injury, bad posture, and particularly as a result of stress, when we hold tension in our muscles.

Treatment Osteopathy treats the whole skeleton, and the muscles and ligaments that hold it together. You will be asked to undress to your underwear and lie in different positions on the treatment couch while the practitioner manipulates and massages the affected muscles and joints, often including the neck, spine, and shoulders, as these are central to skeletal support. It is sometimes uncomfortable, but not usually painful, and the resultant relief from muscular tension is very pleasurable.

Craniosacral work

More than 50 years after the advent of osteopathy a student of Dr. Still's, William Garner Sutherland, developed a technique of manipulating the bones of the skull, which until then had been thought to be one solid structure. Craniosacral work has become particularly popular and successful as a treatment for newborn babies and young children to create body balance, healing, and calm after birth trauma, and for a wide range of symptoms including headache and irritable bowel syndrome.

How does it work? Pressure on the brain from skull misalignment can affect all areas of the body. Tiny, almost imperceptible movements of the eight sections of the

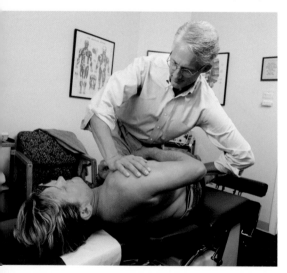

skull can regulate the flow of cerebrospinal fluid, which protects the brain and spinal cord, and release that pressure, along with any tension in the upper neck where the spine meets the skull.

Treatment This is very gentle and soothing; you will barely perceive the movements of the practitioner's hands on your head and neck. It is

Bodily tension can create misalignment of your skeleton. Manipulative therapies can help.

neither frightening nor painful. You will generally feel calm and refreshed after a session, but craniosacral work can sometimes release repressed emotions.

Chiropractic

When he founded the technique of chiropractic in the late 19th century, Dr. Palmer believed, like Still and Sutherland, that displacement of the skeleton caused disease.

How does it work? Chiropractic differs from osteopathy in that chiropractors direct the manipulation primarily to the specific bone or joint, usually in the spine, not to the surrounding muscle. It is very effective for some types of back pain, migraine, sports injuries, and tinnitus, as well as improving asthma and some disorders of the digestive system.

Treatment Chiropractic is like osteopathy, only the manipulations feel sharper and more mechanical. It can be disconcerting to hear your bones click as the joints are flexed at unusual angles, but it is not usually painful.

Bowen Technique

Not a manipulative but a vibrational energy technique, Bowen is a suitable healing therapy for those who are made nervous by the more robust nature of osteopathy. First pioneered by Australian Tom Bowen in the 1950s the technique is very effective where there is chronic muscular pain. It improves joint mobility, promotes the elimination of toxins from the body, and is also said to be helpful in treating a large number of conditions including allergies, asthma, frozen shoulder, and repetitive strain injury (RSI).

How does it work? A qualified Bowen practitioner can detect stress buildup in muscle tissue, and by balancing and stimulating the energy flow through the body, the technique encourages the body to heal itself.

Treatment The Bowen therapist will perform a sequence of light, gentle, precise movements that involve placing the hands on the body through light clothing, but not manipulating it. After the sequence of movements the practitioner pauses to allow the body to respond before continuing with the next sequence. The therapy promotes a deep sense of relaxation.

Massage

Massage is not only a technique for releasing muscle tension, it is also a form of healing through human touch. Rather than an occasional indulgence, massage should be a regular part of any health routine. And if you are feeling anxious, or low in energy, massage can bring a great sense of relaxation and well-being.

How does it work? When the skin and soft tissue are stimulated by touch during massage the flow of oxygen is improved, the lymph glands are stimulated to eliminate toxins such as stress hormones, the muscles relax, and endorphins – the good-mood chemicals – are released. In Eastern massage techniques, the flow of energy, or chi, is said to be unblocked and balanced.

In a world where many of us, especially in the West, do not experience much physical intimacy even in childhood, massage offers a chance to be nurtured in a hands-on way, and as a result some people find it draws strong emotions, such as unresolved grief, to the surface, giving the chance to let them go.

Massage techniques There are many different massage techniques. Some concentrate on muscle relaxing, some on elimination and cleansing, some on unblocking chi, some are holistic, others concentrate on the injured area, but they all promote relaxation and the release of tension. Try a variety of the different massages discussed below to find the one that suits you.

The therapist is as important as the technique. Before treating you, a good therapist will ask about your general health and emotional state, and whether you are taking any medication.

For the best results you will probably need to see the practitioner a number of times, and regularly if possible, so find one you feel completely comfortable with and make sure they are fully qualified, as this is an intimate procedure. Following treatment you may feel tired, and you should drink lots of water to help wash out the toxins released from the tissues during massage.

Shiatsu A holistic therapy, shiatsu is a full-body massage. It originated in Japan in the last century but has its roots in traditional Chinese medicine. Shiatsu is very effective for depression, fatigue, insomnia, migraine, and stress-related conditions.

Treatment Just as an acupuncturist uses needles, the shiatsu therapist uses pressure from the thumbs, fingers, elbows, and knees on the acupoints to release tension and blocked body energy. Longer, more rhythmic strokes over the body are also used. The few seconds when an acupoint is being pressed can be uncomfortable but a skilled therapist will be sensitive to your tolerance.

Swedish massage An invigorating technique, Swedish massage is not holistic and its benefits are short term. The strokes it employs were developed by Per Henrik Ling over 100 years ago as a therapeutic treatment and will be familiar if you have seen anyone being massaged in an old movie! Swedish massage is good for general relaxation and muscle stiffness, especially after exercise.

Treatment The technique includes kneading with thumbs or fingers in a specific spot (petrissage), long, sweeping strokes across the skin (effleurage), and a hacking motion performed in small, fast movements, up and down the body, with the side of the hand or cupped hands (tapotement).

Indian head massage A very different kind of massage, Indian head massage is intensely relaxing and can make you feel quite light-headed and floaty. It has been popular in India for centuries. Benefits include improved concentration, and alleviation of anxiety, tension headaches, and sinusitis.

Treatment The treatment concentrates on the head, face, neck, shoulders, and upper back. It employs a sequence of circular movements across the head using the thumbs, fingers, and hands. A light massage oil is sometimes used.

Hot stones massage Although said to stem from ancient Greece, hot stones is the newest massage idea. Apart from being a very soothing and pleasant experience, hot stones massage is said to boost the circulation and provide an energizing treatment.

Treatment Smooth, flat stones are heated and oiled then placed at strategic points along the body, usually at chakra points, up the spine, in the palms of the hands, and even between the toes. The therapist then uses more hot stones to apply massage strokes to the muscles. During massage, cold stones may be alternated with hot, and the stones are said to be more effective massage tools than the hands.

Posture

The way we hold our bodies, standing and sitting, is important on many levels. Poor posture strains muscles, cramps internal organs, and reduces lung capacity and therefore energy; it also makes us look older and less attractive. If you want to improve your energy, improve your posture.

Young children have perfect posture but, perhaps when we become less comfortable with our bodies as they grow, many of us begin to slouch and slump, then carry these bad habits into adulthood. A misaligned spine can cause havoc.

Beware poor posture Stooped or slumped or round-shouldered means:
■ Back and stomach muscles become weakened.
■ Chest muscles stiffen and shorten, and the spine is no longer properly supported.
■ It becomes difficult to stand up straight for more than a few minutes without effort and the spinal vertebrae and intervertebral disks may be thrown out of alignment.
■ Shoulder muscles become tense and back muscles are forced to compensate, which creates a whole-body tension leading to long-term neck and back problems, tension, and fatigue.
■ The lungs cannot fully expand, so oxygen intake and carbon dioxide output fall leading to loss of energy and retention of toxins.

Posture traps The modern world is full of posture traps. First, our reliance on the car discourages exercise and forces us to sit scrunched up for hours at a time. Next, the increasingly widespread use of computers means we spend more hours at our desks, both at home and at work, hunched in front of a screen that is probably at the wrong height.

Frequent use of the telephone, land lines and mobiles, creates tension up and down the side of the body on which we hold the apparatus, causing compensatory tension on the other side.

Watching TV encourages long hours slumped in an armchair. Air travel now has its own "economy class syndrome" caused by sitting squashed in cheap seats with little leg room as we span the globe. And don't forget high-heeled shoes that, because they tip the body forward, are renowned for throwing women's backs out.

The list, unfortunately, is endless. So how can you save your posture?

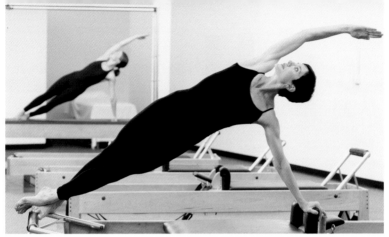

Pilates is an excellent form of exercise for people of any age and fitness.

First steps to good posture In the course of our daily lives there is much we can do ourselves to improve and maintain good posture. Here are a few tips:

- Stand, sit, and walk head up, as if pulled by a string from the top of your head.
- Keep your shoulders down and back; shoulders relaxed, the neck long.
- Do not cross your legs when sitting or standing; this skews the body.
- Go barefoot as much as possible; avoid high-heeled or uncomfortable shoes.
- Ensure that your desk and chair are the right height for your computer. The screen should be at eye level. If you use a laptop, raise the screen on books.
- Get a desk chair that properly supports the small of your back.
- Move around more. Get out of the sitting position at least twice an hour.
- Alternate the hand you use for the phone or mobile.
- Follow proper lifting techniques.
- Keep your weight down.
- Have a regular massage.
- EXERCISE!

Postural therapies

The therapies we discuss here are excellent for realigning the spine and training the body in the habit of good posture. And, if you suffer back problems or experience constant low-level muscle pain, it is worth consulting a reputable posture realignment expert. You will be surprised how much it will change your feeling of well-being and energy levels for the better.

Pilates Over the past five years Pilates has become a hot trend in the exercise world, although Joseph Pilates developed the technique in the 1930s and it has been a well-kept secret among dancers since World War II. Pilates is an excellent exercise system for any age, and is especially useful after injury as it is gentle and offers a large variety of exercises.

How does it work? Pilates focuses on strengthening, toning, and stretching the body. It works the entire body through repetitions of exercises, including a special breathing technique.

Pilates students are encouraged to attune mentally to their body, so they become aware of how each muscle is responding. And by making each movement count, the exercises take less time to become effective. The result is a strong core stability in the body to support the spine and improve posture, flexibility, and balance.

How is it taught? Pilates can be taught in groups or individually. It includes a combination of mat-work and time on the Pilates machines; these work isometrically, meaning the muscles use the machine to work against.

Your technique is constantly monitored by instructors to be sure you are working correctly, and it is possible to progress to a very advanced level if you choose.

Alexander Technique Frederick Matthias Alexander was born in Tasmania in 1869. He became an actor, but when he developed voice problems for which doctors could offer no solution, Alexander set about finding out what he could do for himself.

The technique he developed quickly became internationally popular. The Alexander Technique forms an integral part of many performers' fitness regimes and, like Pilates, it is suitable for people of any age and can be both very calming and empowering.

How does it work? Alexander's system is based on the theory that we misuse our bodies, unconsciously acquiring habits in standing, sitting, and walking that distort the body and interfere with its natural functions, resulting in tiredness, ill health, and muscle pains. He believed that by changing bad habits for good we empower our bodies to function healthily and with energy.

How is it taught? Alexander teachers see themselves as educators. They aim to point out where posture is sabotaging general health and well-being, and to resolve this by teaching new habits and relaxation techniques through gentle manipulation, exercises, and verbal guidance. Alexander classes are taught one-to-one.

During a class, you may seem to do very little, sometimes just quietly lying down or walking around, but all the time you will be learning body awareness and about the correct pattern of movement for your body. The theory is that once your body has relearned these patterns it will automatically apply them to everything you do, from washing up to getting out of a car.

Feldenkrais method Moshe Feldenkrais, a Russian scientist, came to England during World War II. He suffered persistent problems from a knee injury and developed his theory that the patterns for our posture and movement, bad or good, are set in infancy when they are learned, in the same way that we learn language, from our parents.

How does it work? Feldenkrais believed that poor posture and movement could affect our neurological pathways, and our emotional and physical health. His method is designed to create maximum efficiency in body function with the minimum effort.

How is it taught? Feldenkrais is a holistic method of exercise that is taught in two parts: one part is a class called "awareness through movement" and employs a sequence of slow, gentle movements performed while lying on a mat; the other part is called "functional integration," which is taught one-to-one with the teacher using touch and manipulation to correct movements and posture.

Rolfing Founded by Dr. Ida Rolf, an American biochemist, Rolfing is a holistic therapy involving soft-tissue manipulation and movement education. It is said to be very effective in increasing vitality, and in improving posture and balance.

Rolfing is very successful in realigning and relaxing the body. It can also induce a deep emotional response.

How does it work? Rolfing comprises a number of hour-long sessions of deep-tissue massage, which applies strong pressure to a point for two to three seconds at a time.

Sometimes the therapist uses his or her knuckles and elbows to apply pressure, and treatment can be quite painful.

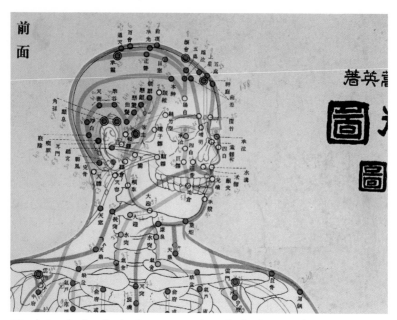

Stimulating the hundreds of acupoints along the body's meridian, or energy, lines can release and balance blocked energy.

The healing arts

Therapies that stimulate and release the flow of energy through the body are beneficial for a multitude of physical and emotional problems including pain relief, weight loss, quitting smoking, and insomnia. They are also a wonderful pick-me-up for those suffering from a general feeling of sluggishness and fatigue.

Acupuncture The ancient technique of acupuncture is perhaps the complementary therapy in which Westerners, including practitioners of conventional medicine, have most faith; many doctors now include acupuncture in treatment. Numerous research studies back up the efficacy of acupuncture, particularly for pain relief. Always consult a fully qualified practitioner.

How does it work? The body has 12 principle meridians, or energy conduits. Each meridian has two channels, one on each side of the body, through which energy, or chi, flows. Meridians are involved in the body's balance of yin and yang; half of the meridians are yin, including the heart, spleen, pancreas, liver, kidneys, lungs, and circulation; and half are yang, including the stomach, large and small intestine, bladder, gallbladder, and what is called the triple heater. Along the meridians lie hundreds of acupoints, and it is these that the acupunture needles stimulate to release and balance blocked energy.

Yin and yang According to Taosim, the spiritual philosophy behind traditional Chinese medicine, everything on earth has its opposing force, represented by yin and yang; there is also yin within yang and vice versa. This duality creates balance without which there would be no life force and which, when it is upset, makes us ill.

Treatment First, the acupuncturist takes a history of your health and emotional state, then diagnoses where the body system is out of balance by checking for various visual clues in the eyes, tongue, and skin, and by taking your pulse.

Depending on the symptoms, fine needles are inserted into a few or many acupoints. You may feel tired or emotional after a treatment and, as the body rebalances, symptoms often worsen before they improve.

Acupressure Based on the same principles as acupuncture and, indeed, thought to predate it, acupressure uses massage techniques instead of needles to stimulate the acupoints – useful if you are needle phobic. It can also be self-administered as a first-aid treatment for pain or minor ailments such as headaches or travel sickness.

Reflexology Forms of reflexology exist in many ancient healing systems, but the modern one stems from the early 20th century when an American, Dr. William Fitzgerald, divided the body into 10 vertical zones across which he allocated the organs. In the 1930s fellow American, Eunice Ingham, believed that the feet mirrored the body and allocated a reflex point on the foot for each body area.

Treatment The feet are massaged with fingers and thumbs to detect granular deposits: lactic acid, calcium crystals, and uric acid. The deposits are said to signal weakness and blockages in different organs, and massaging the reflex points breaks down these deposits, freeing the energy flow to the relevant organ.

The massage pressure can be firm and sometimes painful when a sensitive reflex point is being treated. It is not uncommon to develop a headache and feel tired after treatment as the toxins are being eliminated.

holistic
healing

Complementary therapies are not a quick fix for ill health or low energy. They require commitment to lifestyle changes, and we have to take some responsibility for the way in which the course of our therapy proceeds. Working with an experienced practitioner is an excellent way to find a tailor-made health regime with a good chance of success, and one that can be used either as the sole therapy for a problem, or in conjunction with conventional medicine.

Traditional Chinese medicine

Traditional Chinese medicine (TCM) is one of the most developed healing systems in the world. It dates back thousands of years, but has adapted to the changing face of modern medicine. TCM is still used extensively in China, both in the community and in state hospitals, and encompasses acupuncture, herbal medicine, diet, and exercise disciplines such as tai chi.

Chinese herbal medicine Integral to TCM, Chinese herbal medicine is based on the same philosophy: the balance between yin and yang, and the flow of energy, or qi, within the body. (See "acupuncture" p. 120.) Its uses in the treatment of illness are wide-ranging and include skin, respiratory, and digestive conditions, and chronic fatigue syndrome.

If you suffer low energy for which there seems to be no medical reason, a TCM practitioner may be able to identify the cause of your problem and might prescribe a combination of Chinese herbs and acupuncture to raise your energy level.

Natural preparations Conventional medicine uses drugs based on plants, but there is a big difference between these and herbal medicines. Conventional drugs take the active ingredient out of the plant source, whereas herbal medicine uses the plant in its more natural state, giving greater depth and balance to the preparation.

The active substance in conventional medicines is often prescribed singly, whereas herbal medicines use combinations of herbs that complement each other, giving the remedy a broader but gentler application. Chinese herbs are less likely to cause allergic reactions or the long-term damage associated with some conventional medicines.

Are Chinese herbs safe? All medicines, including herbal preparations, should be treated with respect. Just because a substance is labeled "herbal," does not mean that it can be taken without proper information and supervision. Women who are pregnant or breast-feeding are advised against taking herbal medicines.

Chinese herbs should be prescribed by a qualified practitioner, both to avoid the risk of self-prescription for the wrong condition, and because a reputable practitioner will provide the best quality of herb with correct instructions for its use.

TCM and low energy TCM is a complex healing system, but put very simply, it identifies some of the causes of low energy as a lack of qi, yin, yang, or blood. **Qi** Someone lacking in qi might feel weak and lethargic, almost torpid. Symptoms will vary depending on the area of the body that is unbalanced but a lack of spleen

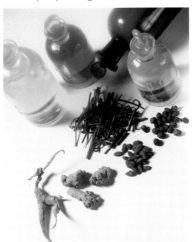

qi, for example, might cause poor appetite and digestion, and frequent diarrhea. The tongue may be pale with tooth-mark serrations and there may be a deep pulse. Herbs that might be given include astragulus (huang qi), codonopsis root (dang shen), and Chinese yam (shan yao). **Yang** This is characterized by fire.

Chinese herbal preparations address all health problems, including low energy levels.

Someone who is yang-deficient might feel tired, very cold, emotionally withdrawn, have a low libido, and might suffer from respiratory problems such as wheezing. Herbs that might be given include gecko (ge jie) and cordyceps fungus (dong chong xia cao).

Yin This is characterized by water. Yin-deficient people are often identified by their high-strung, nervous personalities. They might find it hard to sleep and suffer from dryness and heat, such as a dry cough and night sweats. They have a fast, deep pulse, and a red tongue with hardly any coating. Herbs that might be given include American ginseng root (xi yang shen) and asparagus tuber (tian men dong).

Blood Someone with blood deficiency might feel dizzy, have palpitations, and suffer from vertigo. Their pulse might be threadlike. Herbs that might be given include Chinese angelica root (dang gui) and white peony root (bai shao).

Taking Chinese herbs Most commonly, the TCM practitioner will prescribe a combination of herbs to drink as an infusion after boiling them with water; their bitter taste can take a while to get used to, but some remedies can also be taken in pill form. During treatment, the TCM practitioner will also monitor diet and exercise.

Naturopathy

Natural medicine is holistic in approach and believes that the body is a self-healing organism. Naturopaths do not only aim to heal, they also aim to provide the right environment for the body to heal itself, through education and natural therapies that balance the body systems and boost immune function.

Whole-body health The term "naturopathy" was coined in the late 19th century, but natural medicine has been practiced for hundreds of years. It covers a multitude of disciplines that address whole-body health rather than the symptoms of illness.

The disciplines encompassed by naturopathy include herbalism, nutrition, fasting, cleansing, exercise, fresh air, stress-reduction techniques, hydrotherapy, massage, and bodywork therapies such as osteopathy.

Teaching us to look after ourselves Natural medicine practitioners feel that education is as important as the therapies themselves. The prevention of disease is their aim, and teaching us how to take responsibility for our own health and how to follow a wholesome lifestyle is, they believe, the best way to stimulate and support self-healing.

Naturopaths will search for the underlying cause of major or minor symptoms, rather than treat the symptoms alone. They offer therapies that are noninvasive and do not involve drugs, although many naturopaths now take an integrated approach to health and will support, for example, a cancer patient undergoing chemotherapy, with natural therapies.

Water as therapy

Water promotes well-being; it soothes, relaxes, cleanses, and invigorates us. As a healing treatment it can be applied topically in the form of a compress or wrapping. As a relaxing therapy it can be liquid or steam in the form of steam baths, mineral and seawater spas, hot tubs, sitz baths, and flotation tanks.

Flotation therapy Developed in America in the 1970s, flotation therapy is based on the theory that weightlessness and lack of external stimuli allow the mind and body to relax completely. It is said to reduce anxiety and stress and promote a wonderful sense of mental and physical relaxation. But if you suffer from claustrophobia, this therapy is not for you.

Treatment In a dimly lit room, you are immersed in a tank of warm (body temperature) water that contains mineral salts. Each therapy session lasts up to one-and-a-half hours.

Colonic irrigation Increasingly popular, colonic irrigation is a way of cleansing toxins and increasing energy levels. The theory is that the toxins we inhale and ingest collect in the bowel and, unless they are flushed out, can be absorbed into the bloodstream. So cleansing the colon helps detoxify the whole body.

Colonic irrigation may be beneficial for chronic constipation sufferers who may be feeling sluggish, although improving diet and drinking more water are better long-term solutions.

Treatment Purified water at body temperature is passed gently, via a tube, into the rectum and high up into the colon, then allowed to drain out, taking the bowel contents with it. This is repeated until the water runs clear.

Herbal therapy

Herbs have many uses in supporting health and treating disease (see "Diet" p. 92). The remedies listed below boost immune system function and help with relaxation:

Echinacea (*Echinacea purpurea*) is taken by many as a daily prophylactic against infection; it also increases white cell production and therefore promotes healing.

Goldenseal (*Hydrastis canadensis*) is effective in treating viral infections and also chronic fatigue syndrome. It can be taken with echinacea to treat symptoms.

Cat's claw (*Unicaria tomentosa*) has attracted claims as an antioxidant, antiviral, antiinflammatory, and anticancer agent.

Always consult your doctor before taking any herbal medicines if you are on immunosuppressive drugs, pregnant, or breast-feeding.

Flower remedies and essential oils

Extracting the essence of plants and flowers to use in the treatment of disease dates back to all ancient healing systems; now two 20th-century therapies, aromatherapy and Bach flower remedies, have given the older knowledge a modern resonance.

Bach flower remedies Dr. Bach created his healing remedies in 1920s London. Observing that those of his patients with a positive outlook recovered more quickly, Bach concluded that it was better to treat a patient's state of mind than the disease; sort out emotional conflict, and the body will be able to heal itself.

Energy patterns Flower essence practitioners believe that the energy patterns in plants and flowers correspond to our subtle energy (see p. 106), so they can balance our systems giving us strength to heal ourselves. Fresh flower heads in spring water are left in the sun for three hours; the water takes on the flowers' energy pattern and is then preserved in brandy and stored in dark glass.

The remedies Bach identified 38 plant remedies and divided them into seven main groups of emotions: fear, loneliness, uncertainty, lack of interest in life, overconcern for others, despair, and oversensitivity.

The remedies are safe to self-prescribe and examples include:

Olive for mental and physical exhaustion after a long struggle. **Agrimony** for those who hide internal suffering. **Larch** for low self-esteem and lack of confidence. **Rescue remedy** is a combination of remedies for shock, trauma, or acute anxiety.

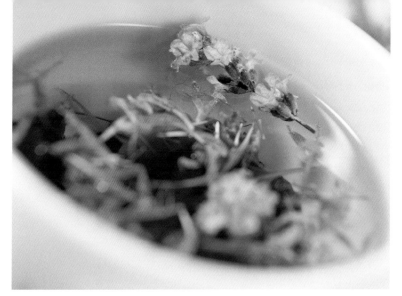

Flower remedies, created by Dr. Bach, treat a patient's state of mind rather than the disease itself.

Aromatherapy Used to reduce stress and tension, balance body energy, support the immune system, and promote a sense of calm and well-being, the modern form of aromatherapy began in 1920s France. Noticing that his burned hand healed rapidly after being dipped in lavender oil Rene Maurice Gattefosse, a chemist, developed the theory that plant essential oils for healing could have a positive effect on the mind as well as being applied directly to a wound.

Treatment Essential oils can be smelled and inhaled, or absorbed through the skin. After taking a history, and before the massage, a therapist will ask you to sniff a few oils to find which feels right for you. We are powerfully affected by smells, and one you dislike will have little benefit even if it is right for the symptoms.

Essential oils Essential oils are extracted from plant material such as bark, flowers, and roots, by various methods including steam distillation and expression. Volatile and powerful, they are blended with a carrier oil such as almond.

The following oils include properties said to promote well-being and calm: **Clary sage** (*Salvia sclarea*) not advised during pregnancy or with alcohol. **Sweet orange** (*Citrus sinensis*) the distilled version can cause sensitivity to light; the expressed version is safe. **Rosewood** (*Aniba rosaeodora*) has no contraindications.

Homeopathy

Homeopathy works on the premise that disease is caused by an imbalance in the body's subtle energy (see p. 106), or "vital force," and that like cures like. By inducing a reaction similar to the disease symptoms, homeopathic remedies activate and support the body's self-healing mechanism; for example, quinine, which is used to treat malaria, triggers malarial symptoms in a healthy person.

More than 2,000 years after Hippocrates put forward the "law of similars" an 18th-century German physician, Dr. Samuel Hahnemann, developed the principle that "like cures like," and called it homeopathy. Hahnemann treated patients with very dilute doses of his remedies, selected in conjunction with his intricate assessment of their symptoms, lifestyle, and general psychological outlook. Today, homeopathy is practiced worldwide to treat a very wide range of conditions.

Assessing "constitution" is fundamental In homeopathic terms "constitution" refers not only to our general state of health but also to temperament, and any inbuilt characteristics; it is the first thing a homeopath will assess.

The homeopathic tincture remedy is "potentized," then added to lactose pilules that dissolve on the tongue.

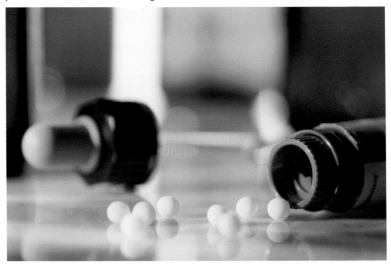

Treatment The assessment of constitution forms the basis for the choice of remedy to treat the symptoms of each individual's disease so, despite having similar symptoms, one person may be prescribed very different remedies to another.

The practitioner will assess everything that affects general well-being, from personality and way of life, to diet and past medical history. The remedies may make you feel worse at first, and future treatment will take account of any reactions.

Potentizing the mother tincture Homeopathic remedies are made from chopped or ground plants or minerals, mixed with alcohol and distilled water. The mixture is left to stand, then strained or pressed to produce the mother tincture. This is then "potentized" by diluting and shaking until the required strength, or potency, is achieved. The remedy is then added to lactose pilules (tiny pills), tablets, granules, or powder and stored in dark glass, or made into ointment or cream.

How to take the remedies Homeopath Dr. Andrew Lockie recommends the following tips to help you get the best from homeopathic remedies:
- Don't touch; drop remedies directly from a clean, dry teaspoon into your mouth.
- Don't eat, or brush your teeth for 30 minutes before or after taking remedies.
- Avoid alcohol, coffee, spicy food, and chemical cleaning agents during treatment.
- Secure tops, and don't return tablets that have been touched to the container.
- Remedies will be more effective if you eat well, exercise, and are free of stress.

Self-medication You can self-prescribe for minor ailments such as colds or insomnia, but always consult your doctor or a qualified homeopath if you are already on medication, for serious conditions, or if symptoms persist. A reputable homeopathic guide, such as Dr. Lockie's *Homeopathy Handbook*, will help with self-assessment and to select remedies for your symptoms.

Tiredness and low energy might be treated by some of the following:

China treats insomnia and exhaustion, good for headaches and indigestion.

Cuprum met helps physical and mental exhaustion, relieves pain, cures cramps.

Antimonium tart reduces exhaustion, relieves pain, heals skin conditions.

Silica heals, strengthens, fights infection, soothes.

Calc carb calms anxiety, eases palpitations, is good for eczema.

Ayurveda

The Indian healing philosophy, Ayurveda, is thought to be the oldest in the world. It is as much a way of life as a healing art, so hopeless if you're looking for a quick fix. Ayurveda believes that a pure, clean body, free from toxins, becomes a temple of creativity, and indomitable spirit.

Mind, body, spirit, balance The word Ayurveda is derived from the Sanskrit meaning "knowledge of daily living," and the philosophy incorporates mind, body, spirit therapies including cleansing and detoxing, nutrition, yoga, meditation, and massage. Based on the same principles as traditional Chinese medicine, Ayurvedic medicine believes that the five elements – earth, water, fire, air, and space – must be balanced within the three bodily humors (the tri-dosha).

The tri-dosha The doshas, called vatta, pitta, and kapha, are present in every living cell. We are made up of all three doshas, but one or two will dominate – you might be kapha, or vatta-pitta, or pitta-kapha.

Find your dosha blueprint Defining your dosha is fundamental to all Ayurvedic treatment. When your doshas are disrupted for any reason – lifestyle, stress, incompatible foods, seasonal changes – your prana (vital life force) is affected, and illness and low energy result.

Vatta represents air and space (ether), and governs motion and breathing. A vatta type will be ectomorph: tall and slim, with lean muscles. They have a fast metabolism and nervous energy, and are quick witted, energetic, restless, and intuitive. They may sleep lightly, tend to be anxious, and lead a creative but erratic existence. Skin and hair are dry and coarse. They walk and talk quickly and are easily excited. They may suffer from constipation and gas.

Diet to balance vatta: sweet, salty, heavy, oily, hot food, such as lentils, brown rice, root vegetables, nuts, honey, chicken, seafood, and orange, yellow, and red fruits.

Pitta represents fire and water and governs digestion and temperature. A pitta type will be mesomorph: medium, athletic build, with broad shoulders and narrow hips. They are strong-minded, intelligent, stubborn, and assertive, with an ordered, perfectionist streak. They are fair with a tendency to freckles. They dislike hot, spicy food, hot weather, too much sun, and they lose their tempers easily.

Diet to balance pitta: sweet, bitter, astringent, cold, heavy, dry food such as chicken, fish, avocado, mango, plums, asparagus, broccoli, white rice, and wheat. **Kapha** represents water and earth and governs stability and energy. A kapha type will be endomorph: large, fleshy, heavy build, with short legs and arms. They are strong, caring, and calm, with good stamina, and a tendency to fat. They have a good memory, need a lot of sleep, move slowly, and won't be rushed. They have a tendency to excess mucus production and dislike damp weather.

Diet to balance kapha: pungent, bitter, astringent, light, dry, hot food, such as chilies, apples, cranberries, dried fruit, beets, cabbage, shrimp, and turkey.

Panchakarma This group of therapies tackles the cleansing and detoxifying element in Ayurveda. The cleansing process begins with snehan, a detoxifying massage done with oil, and swedan, purification through steam baths, which often includes the use of detoxifying herbs. Other cleansing rituals follow including:

■ Therapeutic vomiting after drinking licorice or salt water.
■ Purging with laxatives, such as senna.
■ Enemas.
■ Nasal massage and nasal washes with medicated powder or liquid.
■ Blood purification with herbal detoxifiers such as burdock root tea.

Marma therapy This is a massage therapy designed to relieve stress-related illness, heal injuries, and energize the body by balancing the tri-dosha. Warm, medicated oils are applied generously during a full-body massage, concentrating on the marmas (energy points) in the body. There are said to be 107 marmas, and that these are the junctions of the five "principles" – flesh, veins, arteries, tendons, and bones and joints.

Ayurveda is a way of life If you are interested in how your dosha type affects your choice of exercise and diet, you need to consult a practitioner.

Ayurveda is a very complex health philosophy and to derive full benefit it should be embraced as a whole, not just picking a therapy here and there. Done properly, Ayurveda requires a complete change in the way you live and it does take considerable commitment.

Therapies based on vibrations

Everything in the universe is made up of vibrational energy, which vibrates at different frequencies to create color, light, and sound; think of rainbows, crystals, and music. It is thought by some that these vibrational frequencies may have the power to harmonize our own subtle energy (see p. 106) and promote well-being.

Seasonal affective disorder Sunlight makes us feel energized and happy; it stimulates the pineal gland to produce serotonin, the chemical that lifts mood, and can also increase levels of melatonin, the hormone that controls sleep.

Too little serotonin or too much melatonin can lead to depression, drowsiness, and sluggishness, and it is this imbalance that, during winter, can cause seasonal affective disorder, or SAD (see p. 75) in susceptible individuals.

Light therapy Full-spectrum, ultraviolet filtered light mimics natural sunlight and exposing a SAD sufferer to light at a minimum of 2,500 lux via lamps or a light box will usually treat the condition successfully. Sessions, with a therapist, under lights may last up to two hours, then a light box is used at home for up to 20 minutes daily. Light therapy is also used to treat skin conditions, menopausal problems, premenstrual syndrome, and to boost the immune system.

Color and energy We tend to be drawn instinctively to particular colors when choosing which clothes to wear, how we decorate our homes, and in the flowers we like. Color therapists believe that we are drawn to a particular color because we need it to right or maintain our body-energy balance, like a nicotine addict reaching for another cigarette.

We feel more at ease when the color around us harmonizes with our mood. Feeling angry and agitated in a predominately red room unsettles us even more, because red stimulates and excites; turquoise or blue are soothing.

A color therapist might begin by reading your aura – the vibrational energy that some people believe surrounds each of us. Disease and blocked energy are said to show up in dull, dark patches, the colors of health are said to glow.

Color therapists also dowse, holding a crystal pendulum over the chakras (see p. 106), to determine the state of a person's vibrational energy.

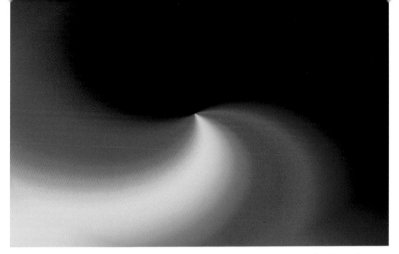

The colors of the rainbow are present in all vibrational energy healing, from crystals to color therapy.

Chakras are represented by the colors of the rainbow, and as crystals emit vibrations of the rainbow spectrum they are thought to interact. The appropriate crystal placed on a chakra can release blocked energy and bring about healing.

Color therapy Therapists use different techniques that bring healing color to the body. Foremost is chromotherapy, or colored light. After diagnosis, the therapist will bathe you, or the affected area, in the appropriate colored light or lights. Advice is also given about the colors with which to surround yourself.

Learn the language of color In her book *New Colour Healing*, Lilian Verner-Bond writes that by learning the language of color we can encourage self-awareness. Each color has a polarity, and positive and negative aspects.

Green polarity is balance and imbalance. Positive aspects include tact, discrimination, stability, generosity, imagination, reform, and lack of bias; negative aspects include jealousy, resentfulness, forgetfulness, selfishness, and greed.

Gold polarity is trust and deception. Positive aspects include generosity, maturity, wisdom, vitality, forgiveness, triumph, and experience; negative aspects include suspicion, paranoia, pessimism, conceit, disgrace, and underachievement.

Orange polarity is activity and laziness. Positive aspects include strength, untiring energy, fearlessness, freedom, justice, tolerance, and a warm heart; negative aspects include being overbearing, pessimistic, self-indulgent, and an exhibitionist.

Positive thinking

We are how we think. Pessimists find the world a miserable place, and many of us do not realize just how negatively we see ourselves and others, and how much this affects every aspect of our life. Positive thinking vastly improves health and energy.

The Victor Meldrew syndrome We laugh at this miserable old man in T.V.'s *One Foot in the Grave.* He's always complaining; nothing is ever right. And he believes it, so nothing *is* ever right. But we do it too: "I can't do that," "I'm not worth that," "He won't look at me," "I'm hopeless at...."

According to ancient philosophies such as vipassana and vedanta, and modern psychological disciplines including cognitive therapy and neurolinguistic programming (NLP) (see p. 137), feelings of inadequacy are self-perpetuating. If you believe you're a failure, you will fail. The solution is simple; change your thought patterns and you can change your life.

Affirm the positive Affirmations work on the principle of recognizing god or the universal spirit within ourselves. If you believe you are full of goodness and love,

Laughter increases the production of mood-enhancing endorphins and raises oxygen levels.

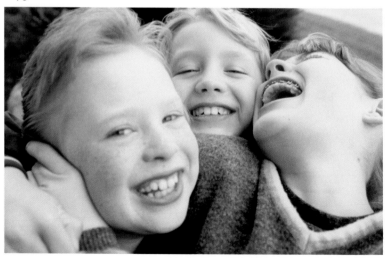

then you will be; you are only recognizing what is already there. Constantly affirming the positive in yourself restores confidence and well-being.

Affirmation techniques Affirmations are very powerful, so be clear about your goals and realistic about what you ask for; you might just get it.

Technique 1 Write a list of the things you want to change about yourself, but write it as if they were already true, which, remember, they are, but you haven't recognized it yet. For example, you might write: "I am a successful person who is trusted and valued, and I love myself for who I am and how I look. I deserve this; may I be well and happy."

Check your list to make sure it is what you really want to say, then memorize it and repeat it to yourself, aloud or silently, in groups of seven. Ignore the internal voice telling you it isn't true. Do this as often as you remember – on the bus, at work, before you go to sleep – and within a few weeks your mind pattern will be changing for the better. When one affirmation becomes real, create another.

Technique 2 This is based on an NLP technique. Visualize a negative phrase you always use about yourself, such as "I always make a mess of things" or "No one will ever love me," and watch it fade away into the distance, float up into the sky, gradually getting smaller and smaller, and eventually disappearing. And in its place, coming toward you is the positive version: "I am good at doing things," "I am loved," getting bigger and bigger until it becomes part of you. Or do the same exercise with sound, listening to the negative phrase getting softer at the same time as the positive one gets louder.

Laughter therapy Try some healing laughter; it's a quick, easy, energy buzz. Laughter increases the production of mood-enhancing endorphins and raises oxygen levels. It releases tension, reduces anxiety, and boosts the immune system.

American psychologist and laughter therapist Mariana Funes says that we don't laugh only because we find something funny, but also when we are embarrassed, shy, upset, nervous, and tense. It is an automatic body function like crying or yawning. She suggests a laughter workout where you find a partner and try laughing – for no reason at all – for at least one minute. Don't laugh at anything or anyone, just let go and laugh out loud. You'll feel great.

Talking therapies

Persistent low energy often results from unresolved emotional issues. Most commonly these stem from childhood, but they may be more recent traumas that we find too difficult to talk about. But repress painful thoughts and feelings, and you store up trouble because repression leads to stress, and stress, we know, depletes energy.

Don't bottle up problems The old adage "a problem shared is a problem halved" is absolutely true. But we tend to think that we can solve our own problems, or that it is unfair to burden others with them, or we may be too ashamed to speak about them. Internalizing worry puts us at risk of anxiety and stress.

Most people are only too happy to listen and help, and talking about worries gives them valuable perspective. If you don't feel comfortable talking to a friend, talk to your doctor, or find a counselor. But whatever you do, talk.

Comfort in being heard Sometimes we may be aware of a deeper emotional unhappiness that goes beyond a worry. Our patterns of thinking and how we see ourselves are set in childhood, and people brought up by carertakers who were unable to give enough love and respect might become insecure and lacking in self-esteem.

It is not always easy to open up to a therapist, but the experience for most people is comfort in finally being heard, even if some of the issues are painful to confront. And the end result of knowing yourself better is less anxiety, more confidence, and a calmer mind.

There are many therapies and therapists to chose from. Without getting too New Agey about it, it seems that when we are really ready for therapy we do find the right person to help us; it might be by word of mouth, through a professional body, or by asking your doctor.

You will know from the introductory session whether you feel comfortable enough to trust this person with your thoughts and feelings. If for any reason you are unsure, then look for someone else.

Cognitive behavioral therapy (CBT) American psychoanalyst, Aaron Beck, developed CBT during the 1970s. Successful in the treatment of low self-esteem, and mild to moderate depression, CBT is based on the belief that the key to reducing our neuroses is not exposing past trauma, but instead changing the negative thought patterns caused by that trauma, as it is these thought patterns that have affected our emotions and, ultimately, our behavior.

CBT addresses how we feel and behave in everyday incidents and relationships with others by pinpointing our distorted thought patterns and the ways in which they are affecting our life, then offering alternative ways that we can see ourselves and so generate different, healthier, reactions.

The therapy is usually short term and would typically involve between 10 and 20 structured, goal-oriented sessions.

Psychoanalysis There are many different forms of psychoanalysis, the two main proponents of the therapy being Freud and Jung. Psychotherapists believe that the answers to a dysfunctional or neurotic mind-set lie within the individual's subconscious, where the traumas of childhood are buried. The analyst works with the patient to discover how past traumas are affecting the patient's present life. Psychotherapy can be long term with up to five, 50-minute sessions each week.

Neurolinguistic programming (NLP) A form of psychotherapy, NLP was developed in the 1970s. It believes that by changing our self-image and the way we think, we can free up our emotions and make life work more successfully for us.

NLP involves interaction between therapist and client. To get to the root of the problem, the therapist watches the client's body language, eye movements, breathing, the way he describes his feelings, the way he speaks, and the words he chooses. Then, as with CBT, the therapist teaches ways to rethink attitudes and perceptions, and replace the negative thought patterns that are sabotaging the client's life.

Counseling Counseling is usually a more short-term and less in-depth form of therapy than psychotherapy. It often focuses on a recent trauma, such as bereavement or divorce.

You might see a counselor once a week for up to six months. Counseling provides a safe space in which to air concerns, with someone who will protect your privacy and can help to shed light on problems.

conventional
medicine

At the frontline of conventional medical healthcare in the United States is primary care. Knowing how to use this service and how to take full advantage of all its benefits is vital, not only for treating disease, but also for maintaining health through education and screening.

What general practice offers

Your general practice, of which 90 percent in the U.S. are group practices, offers primary health care. The personnel involved at this level of care include general practitioners (GPs), nurse practitioners, health visitors, community nurses, and midwives, and allied to the practice, physiotherapists and podiatrists, and increasingly complementary therapists – all of whom have a role in modern health education.

This means it is the first point of access for all conventional medical services, including treatment if your doctor is puzzled about the source of your low energy levels.

Understand your treatment Doctors are human like the rest of us, but many people are still overawed by the medical profession and afraid to ask questions, with the result that their treatment may be compromised.

Never allow a doctor to treat you unless you understand what is being done and why, and all the possible outcomes. Don't be afraid to ask questions, and check your doctor's level of competence and expertise by asking for details of his professional record from hospital management or the local medical society.

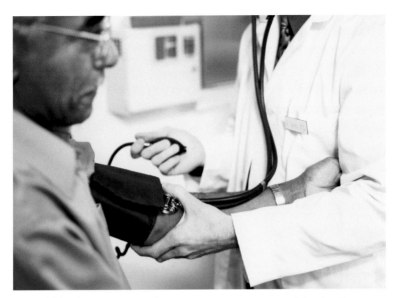

Normal blood pressure is vital to maintaining an energetic lifestyle. Your doctor can measure your blood pressure easily in his office.

Making the most of your GP

Properly explaining a health problem and receiving appropriate advice in the time allocated for GP appointments is not always easy. The following tips will help:

■ Find a GP who really listens to you and who shares your views about treatment options, such as use of antibiotics or complementary medicine. If you have a preference for a male or a female GP, say so.

■ Write brief headings for what you want to tell your GP before your appointment.

■ Tell your GP everything, don't hold back information because it might be embarrassing. They've seen it all!

■ If you think your problem is a difficult one, book two consecutive appointments.

■ Don't waste your GP's time; cancel appointments you can't keep or no longer need, don't call out a doctor without good reason, and if in doubt about the seriousness of your ailment, ask to speak to the practice nurse.

■ Educate yourself about your condition – the Internet is good information source.

■ Take responsibility for your day-to-day health. Prevention is better than cure.

Screening and tests

Always attend screening appointments as they are the first line of defense against cancers.

Tests your GP might order include pulse, blood pressure and heart monitoring, and taking samples, such as blood or urine, for analysis. If you are referred to a hospital for tests, your GP will monitor the results and may be the one who will initiate treatment.

We are advised to have dental checkups at least once a year, particularly as a link has been found between gum disease and heart disease, and those over 45 should have their eyes tested annually for glaucoma (abnormally high fluid pressure inside the eye).

Blood pressure measurement This is to check that your blood pressure is not too high, risking heart disease and stroke. It should be checked every five years after the age of twenty for both women and men, and your GP will test this.

Pap smear test This tests for cancer of the cervix, or precancerous changes in cervical cells. Women in the U.S. should have a smear test every two years from the start of sexual activity onward, and more frequently if abnormal cells have been detected. Your GP or nurse practitioner will perform this procedure, or it can be done in a family planning clinic or womens' health center.

Mammogram This is to test for breast cancer and involves a simple X-ray of the breasts. In the U.S. it is recommended every three years beginning at age 40; at age 50 it is recommended annually.

Bone density This is used to detect osteoporosis in women and is advised every few years beginning at age 40.

Sigmoidoscopy This is a scan for colon cancer and is recommended at age 50 and at five-year intervals thereafter.

organizations

Acupuncture

American Association of

Acupuncture and Oriental

Medicine

1424 16th Street NW, Suite 501

Washington DC 20036

www.aaaom.org

Herbalism

American Holistic Medical

Association

6728 Old McLean Village Drive

McLean, Virginia 22101

www.holisticmedicine.org

Homeopathy

American Institute of Homeopathy

1585 Glencoe

Denver, Colorado 80220

Tel: 303-370-9164

www.homeopathyusa.org

Osteopathy

American Academy of Osteopathy

3500 DePauw Boulevard, Suite 1080

Indianapolis, Indiana 46268-139

Tel: 317-879-0563

www.academyofosteopathy.org

Meditation and Yoga

International Association of

Yoga Therapists

109 Hillside Avenue

Mill Valley, California 94941

www.iayt.org

Massage

Association of Bodyworkers and

Massage Professionals

28677 Buffalow Park Road

Evergreen, Colorado 80439

www.abmp.com

Psychology

American Psychological

Association

750 First Street NE

Washington, DC 20002

Tel: 415-327-2066

www.apa.org

Pain

American Pain Foundation

201 N. Charles Street, Suite 710

Baltimore, Maryland 21201-4111

Tel: 1-888-615-PAIN (7246)

Email: info@painfoundation.org

Allergies

American Academy of Allergy,

Asthma, and Immunology

611 East Wells Street

Milwaukee, WI 53202

Tel:800-822-2762

www.aaaai.org

Diabetes

National Institute of Diabetes and

Digestive and Kidney Diseases

31 Center Drive, MSC2560,

Building 31, Room 9A-04

Bethesda MD 20892-2560

Tel: 800-860-8747

www.niddk.nih.gov/

Nutrition

Food and Nutrition Information

Center

Agricultural Research Service, USDA,

National Agricultural Library,

Room 105

10301 Baltimore Avenue

Beltsville, MD 20705-2351

Tel: 301-504-5719

www.nal.usda.gov/fnic

Sleep

American Sleep Disorders

Association

www.asda.org

index